THE GREAT HUMAN DIGNITY HEIST

How bioethicists are trashing the foundations of Western civilization

Michael Cook

Connor Court Publishing

Published in 2017 by Connor Court Publishing

Copyright © Michael Cook

All rights reserved. No part of this book may be reproduced or transmitted in any form or by any means, electronic or mechanical, including photocopying, recording or by any information storage and retrieval system, without prior permission in writing from the publisher.

Connor Court Publishing Pty Ltd
PO Box 7257
Redland Bay QLD 4165
sales@connorcourt.com

www.connorcourt.com

Phone 0497 900 685

ISBN: 978-1-925501-46-9

Cover design, Maria Giordano

Printed in Australia

For Mom and Pop

Michael Cook likes bad puns, bushwalking and black coffee. He did a BA at Harvard University in the United States where it was good for networking, but moved to Sydney where it wasn't. He also did a PhD on an obscure corner of Australian literature. He has worked as a book editor and a magazine editor and has published articles in magazines and newspapers in the US, the UK and Australia. Currently he is the editor of BioEdge, a newsletter about bioethics, and MercatorNet. He also writes a bioethics column for Australasian Science and contributes occasional op-ed pieces to newspapers and websites in the US, UK and Australia.

MercatorNet is an online magazine with a focus on human dignity.

www.mercatornet.com

BioEdge is a weekly online bioethics newsletter. It covers issues ranging from surrogacy and euthanasia to organ transplants and conscientious objection. One leading progressive bioethicist has acknowledged that BioEdge has "a larger real-world impact than most bioethics journals could dream of".

www.bioedge.org

CONTENTS

Foreword	7
Part 1: Slip Slidin' Away	9
Part 2: Dicing with human dignity	33
Part 3: War heroes	52
Part 4: The miserabilists	75
Part 5: Torture and other utilitarian games	99
Part 6: The reproductive revolution	122
Part 7: Doctors at work	151
Part 8: Homo sapiens 2.0	167
Part 9: Grey matter	179
Part 10: Remember the great stem cell debate?	197
Part 11: Reporting bioethics news	212
Part 12: Peering into the future	237

FOREWORD

We have begun the 21st Century with no reliable moral compass. Many people have lost their connection with traditional religion; schools and universities are reluctant to impart absolute rights and wrongs. What most of us navigate by is a lodestone whose needle swings wildly with our emotions, opinion polls and newspaper op-eds. But social and technological change forces us to confront urgent questions about life, death, birth, sexuality, our bodies, and what it means to be a person.

More and more, politicians, the media, doctors, scientists and the public have turned to professional bioethicists for answers about how to chart their way through these stormy waters. There are probably thousands of academic bioethicists in the United States, and thousands more who "do" bioethics. Every hospital has at least one bioethics committee. Universities and government departments have more committees. Universities now offer degrees in bioethics. The media turn to qualified bioethicists for guidance about how to approach bizarre and unforeseen ways that medicine and technology sometimes touch our lives.

This is understandable. Most of us are unaccustomed to moral and philosophical reasoning. But what gives "bioethicists" authority to pronounce on moral issues? Why are their conclusions more solidly grounded than yours – or your grandmother's or a reader of Tarot cards? Perhaps it has something to do with the name. That sexy little prefix "bio" has become a Kevlar vest for so-called experts who couldn't score a job in the philosophy department of Monty Python's University of Woolloomooloo. Despite its prestige, there is no agreement on what bioethics is, on what areas it should cover, or, most importantly, on its fundamental principles. Just about anyone can dub themselves a bioethicist – and just about anyone does.

The word "bioethics" was only coined in the late 1960s. Forty years on, we have progressive bioethics, conservative bioethics, global bioethics, feminist bioethics, Islamic bioethics, Catholic bioethics, utilitarian bioethics, deontological bioethics, dignitarian bioethics (my favourite), and so on. Bioethics, as most of the real experts quietly agree, is a field in crisis. Some of its leading practitioners have spoken of "a crisis of identity" and have even questioned "the survival of bioethics as we have known it". "Hardly wet behind the ears, bioethics seems destined for a short lifespan," one medical historian has written.

The chaotic state of bioethics is what has encouraged me to contribute to the debate. I am just a journalist; I have no qualifications in bioethics, other than closely observing developments for several years as editor of an online newsletter about bioethics, *BioEdge*. So I come to the field as a layman equipped with facts, common sense, a strong belief in human dignity, and enough cheek to question the self-confident facade of the professionals.

As medicine and technology progress, we need answers to the ethical, social, legal, philosophical dilemmas they create. So we will always need bioethics and bioethicists. But we cannot delegate our future to them. We have to think things through for ourselves. That's what I have done in the brief essays in this book, which have been selected from my contributions over the years to a number of newspapers and magazines in Australia, the United States and Britain. I hope they encourage you to question the "experts".

Part 1
Slip Slidin' Away

The great human dignity heist

I don't think that any other bioethical issue raises more passions than euthanasia. I have always opposed it, although I've tried to recognise the painful situations which drive people to consider it. But I have become used to receiving abusive messages from people who interpret my words as an assault on their integrity. I remember that one of them was: "I hope you die a painful and lingering death from cancer with no prospect of release."

What accounts for the intensity of this feeling? Yes, people everywhere are afraid of pain. But advances in palliative care have made intractable pain rare. What people fear more than pain is lack of autonomy. We live in a culture in which many people feel that dependence is the greatest possible humiliation, whether one has to seek support from a divine power or just from a visiting nurse. I've always seen things differently. Dependence is part of what makes us human. Absolute independence is an illusion which comforts our vanity. In reality we are bound to family, friends, neighbours, our nation and even our ancestors by a web of relationships which have sustained us for our whole lives. "No man is an island, entire of itself; every man is a piece of the continent," as the poet John Donne wrote long ago. But because this sense is so deeply ingrained, we are not likely to see the end of this debate any time soon.

Belgium and the majesty of the law

MercatorNet, 5 January 2014

It appears that Belgian doctors are simply ignoring the clear letter of the law in their zeal to pursue euthanasia.

What was it Winston Churchill said about Russia: "a riddle wrapped in a mystery inside an enigma"? With respect to social policy, much the same applies to Belgium. Supporters of euthanasia there just roll their eyes in exasperation when critics in the English-speaking world thunder about slippery slopes or violations of human dignity.

The two sides are simply failing to mesh gears in the moral debate. The best example of this is a conversation in the leading Belgian newspaper De Standaard between Wim Distelmans and Marc Cosyns, two leading advocates of legalised euthanasia.

Dr Distelmans is the best-known spokesman for euthanasia in Belgium, its best-known practitioner, and the chairman of the Federal Control and Assessment Commission since it was legalised in 2002. Belgian doctors are required to submit a report on every case of euthanasia and submit it to this commission to check that all the statutory procedures have been faithfully followed. If anyone is responsible for ensuring that the legal safeguards are applied rigorously, it is Wim Distelmans.

Dr Cosyns is a palliative care specialist whose views on euthanasia are far more advanced than Distelmans's. He favours the complete decriminalisation of euthanasia so that it will be regarded simply as just another option for palliative care physicians.

This is the background to an astonishing admission made by Dr Cosyns in the course of their conversation. The journalist from De Standaard asked whether he reports the deaths he has caused through euthanasia to the Commission.

"No, not when it comes to our own patients," Dr Cosyns responded. "Everything I do is done on the basis of the law of patients' rights. We should not be required to give assurances that we did not intend to harm the person. Euthanasia is a normal medical procedure, as normal as the possibility of palliative sedation."

In other words, Dr Cosyns, exasperated that Belgium's law does not coincide with his own philosophy of euthanasia, admitted that he ignores it. *The law be damned* is his motto.

Even within the permissive framework of Belgian legislation, Dr Cosyns has clearly committed a crime. He has killed Belgian citizens. He is allowed to do this in those exceptional cases which are defined as euthanasia, but he has refused to report these acts, as he is required to do and as the public expects him to do.

Even Wim Distelmans appeared to be bug-eyed in amazement at this admission. "But Marc," he said gently, "you cannot ignore the criminal law."

So what happened after the publication of the article? A leading public figure confessed to a crime – possibly many crimes – before witnesses who included the "judge" in charge of administering the law for this particular crime. Surely there must have been outrage at the arrogance of a doctor who regards himself as above the law. Surely the head of the commission must have initiated an investigation.

But nothing happened. Nothing at all.

To illustrate just how different things are across the Channel, consider the recent case of Ray Gosling. Gosling was a talented BBC broadcaster and gay rights activist. In 2010 he decided to make a series about death and he interviewed people involved in mercy killings. Then, on the February 15 episode of the BBC magazine show Inside Out, he declared that 16 years ago he himself had smothered an unnamed lover as he lay dying of AIDS to spare him terrible pain.

Now in England there is a lot of sympathy for assisted suicide and mercy killing, particularly amongst the intelligentsia. Nonetheless, it is clearly against the law. The police reacted immediately. Thirty-six hours after the program aired, Gosling was arrested on suspicion of murder. He was released on bail and a six-month investigation ensued.

The police eventually discovered that Gosling had fabricated the whole story and he was given a six-month suspended sentence for wasting police time. (Gosling died in November at the age of 74.)

Why was Gosling arrested while Cosyns is still at large, free to administer lethal injections, accountable to no one except himself? In this juxtaposition lies the difference between the Anglosphere and Belgium.

What can explain it? Is it a white coat exemption, which places doctors and scientists on a pedestal above laws written for patients? Is it a disdain for Europe's Christian heritage so bitter that whatever Christians have condemned must now be condoned?

Or is it an Olympian nonchalance toward "the majesty of the law", the feeling that laws are written for the little people, not the haut monde of people with media profiles and PhDs? If this is the case, foreign observers must be forgiven if they ask whether there will ever be enough safeguards in Belgium's euthanasia legislation to protect the weak, elderly and vulnerable.

The ultimate Christmas present

MercatorNet, 17 December 2004

Santa came early for good little girls and boys in the Netherlands, bringing the gift of involuntary euthanasia for children under 12.

Merry Christmas! From the Netherlands, the country that brought you Santa Claus, comes the ultimate Christmas present, involuntary euthanasia for kids! Groningen Academic Hospital has asked the Dutch government to approve protocols for killing deformed and terminally ill children – after admitting that it had already done this four times in the past year.

The leading figure in the push for "mercy killing" for children, Dr Eduard Verhagen, said that the number affected by the measure would be no more than about a dozen each year. The newborns he has in mind suffer "agonising pain", he said. "The parents watch this in tears and beg the doctor to bring an end to such suffering." His press release failed to mention that the "Groningen protocols" would allow doctors to kill children up to the age of 12, not just infants.

Together with Dutch public prosecutors, Dr Verhagen and his colleagues have drawn up a list of five criteria: "the suffering must be so severe that the newborn has no prospects of a future; there is no possibility of a cure or alleviation with medication or surgery; the parents must always give their consent; a second opinion must be provided by an independent doctor who has not been involved with the child's treatment; and the deliberate ending of life must be meticulously carried out with the emphasis on aftercare."

Dutch doctors want to expand the boundaries of euthanasia to include adults who are sick and tired of living and not just sick.

Santa Claus came for Dutch grown-ups, too. In a separate development, the Dutch medical profession announced that it wants to expand the boundaries of euthanasia to include adults who are sick and tired of living and not just sick. Earlier this month, shortly after the Netherlands Supreme Court upheld the conviction of Dr Philip Sutorius for euthanasia in 1998, the Dutch doctors' association, the KNMG, demanded that the goalposts be shifted. Dr Sutorius had killed an 86-year-old former senator, Edward Brongersma, who had no one to care for him and was tired of living. Perhaps he had reason to be: Brongersma was an outspoken advocate of paedophilia and author of a two-volume study called *Loving Boys*. After spending time in jail for child sex, he became chairman of the Judiciary Committee of the Dutch Senate from 1969 to 1977 and helped to push through repeal of the laws under which he had been convicted.

The KNMG has now released a lengthy report in support of voluntary euthanasia for existential rather than for medical reasons. The chairman of the committee, Dr Jos Dijkhuis, argues that "suffering is too often linked to illness" and that a person who simply cannot bear to live any longer and whose outlook on the future is hopeless is "suffering from life".

None of this comes as a surprise. Dutch doctors have been killing their patients upon request for years with the connivance of the government, even before the practice was legalised in 2002. Immediately thereafter came reports that many doctors were killing patients outside of the agreed guidelines because there was too much red tape. Broadening the ambit of euthanasia to include children under 12 who cannot give informed consent and people whom no medicine can cure because they are not sick is a natural development. Dementia is already deemed a valid reason for euthanasia. As well, it is already an option for 12-year-olds who have their parents' consent.

These Christmas goodies confirm that the Dutch medical profession – with many honourable exceptions -- is suffering from terminal case of navel-gazing.

Doesn't it ask how other countries view Holland's accelerating ride down the slippery slope?

Consider, for instance, what the United States will think. Effectively the Dutch have legalised the death penalty for people whose crime is simply to be young and sick or old and depressed. And this comes from a country which has been wagging its finger at the United States about the immorality of enforcing the death penalty for the mentally ill!

Under the presidency of the Netherlands, the European Commission chided the US for refusing to sign an international agreement banning the execution of people with mental disorders. "The EU restates its firm conviction," it said, "that the execution of persons suffering from mental disorder is contrary to widely accepted human rights norms and standard... In cases where the death penalty is carried out, any miscarriage of justice, which is occasionally inevitable in any legal system, would be irreversible." Euthanasia is also irreversible, but it happens every day in Dutch nursing homes. In 2003 there were 1,815 reported cases of euthanasia, a figure which everyone agrees is greatly understated. In the United States, for all its faults, at least we know how many people are executed every year. In the Netherlands, reliable statistics are unavailable for matters as basic as numbers those killed and their ages.

Consider, too, what Dutch Muslims will think – especially after the brutal murder of a Dutch film-maker for insulting Islam. "Euthanasia violates the purpose of preserving religion, *hifdh ad-din*, because it involves a human attempt to violate the divine prerogative of giving and taking away life," according to the "fatwa bank" of IslamOnline. If many Christians are incensed by the legalisation of euthanasia, what will unbalanced Muslim extremists think? Will it increase their esteem for Dutch culture to know that the test case for the introduction of euthanasia without illness centred on a world-renowned paedophile? Will they admire a relaxed, tolerant, freedom-loving culture which allows involuntary euthanasia of children under 12?

Why the Netherlands has become the epicentre of world euthanasia baffles scholars. But surely one reason is the arrogant assumption that, unless proven otherwise, doctors are rational, well-balanced and compassionate -- ideally suited to decide whether their patients should live or die.

However, doctors may actually be less healthy psychologically than the rest of the population, not more. An Australian review of doctors' emotional health based on international research found that depression, burn-out and psychiatric illness are very common amongst doctors, but few seek professional assistance. They are twice as likely to commit suicide. Female doctors are six times more likely. One study has suggested that doctors were more afraid of death than seriously ill patients. Psychiatrists have the highest suicide rate of all specialties. Giving stressed, depressed and burnt-out doctors the authority to kill their patients, turning a blind eye as they kill without permission, and changing the law when they flout it will eventually lead to abuses on a colossal scale.

It has become clear that the Dutch government and medical

profession have no intention of stopping their country's slide into abuses of the most fundamental of all human rights. It is hypocritical for the Netherlands to demand that countries like Turkey scrub up their record on human rights before applying for membership in the European Union. What the international community must do is apply pressure on the Netherlands to halt its slide down the slippery slope.

Is death really better than disability?
*MercatorN*et, 11 January 2010

Whom better to ask than the disabled? They give some surprising answers.

When assisted suicide is legalised most of the people who will die will be disabled. And American disability advocates take a very dim view of it. This is the theme of a hard-hitting series of articles in the latest issue of the Disability and Health Journal.

The editor, Suzanne McDermott, of the University of South Carolina School of Medicine, writes that she changed her own mind after studying the issue. At first she believed that assisted suicide was solely a personal autonomy issue. But eventually she was persuaded that it is at the heart of the movement for disability rights: "Almost all people at the end of life can be included in the definition of 'disability'. Thus, the practice of assisted suicide results in death for people with disabilities."

The special issue is a response to a controversial 2008 decision by the American Public Health Association (APHA) to back "aid in dying" (ie, assisted suicide). This slipped almost completely under the media's radar, but it means that the official policy of the "oldest, largest and most diverse organization of public health professionals in the world" – 30,000 of them – is to support assisted suicide to the hilt. Or, as they prefer to call it in Oregon, "patient-directed dying" or "physician aid-in-dying".

Rather than worrying about some ambiguous language in the Obama administration's health reform legislation or scrutinising the publications of his health advisors for a few indiscreet phrases, the elderly and their relatives ought to be worried about the 30,000 members of the APHA. They are the ones who could be sitting on the "death panels". The authors of the articles in the *Disability and Health Journal* certainly are worried.

Several themes emerge from the articles.

First, the very existence of legalised assisted suicide leads to an expectation that the disabled, elderly and infirm should shuffle off their mortal coil a bit early to relieve the burden on their carers.

This fear has been ridiculed by supporters, who contend that all they want is choice at the end of life and that a lifelong experience of disability is different from the pain of seeing one's life ebb away. They think that disability advocates are demonising euthanasia lobby groups and exaggerating their own vulnerability

Nonsense, says Diane Coleman, of the lobby group Not Dead Yet. She points out – quite eloquently -- that pity can be more dangerous than a mad doctor in a nursing home. We are, she says, "more frightened by the doctors who are out to help us but who see our lives as burdensome and who know little about options that make life with disability valuable."

Why should valuable resources be wasted on them, anyway? "Every week, I hear another person with a disability recount a disturbing interaction with a physician, nurse, or other health professional who clearly transmitted the view that life with a disability is inherently burdensome," she writes. "It does not feel safe to have one's life in the hands of someone who views that life as unfortunate, maybe even tragic or unfair."

Second, advocates of assisted suicide and euthanasia ignore the experience of the disabled because they think that a dying 80-year-old is radically different from someone who has spent a lifetime in a wheelchair. Show me the evidence for this, Ms Coleman demands. Anyone, at any age, can learn to cope with disability. "To dismiss these efforts as futile because the individual is near the end of life has no empirical foundation and raises questions about the commitment of assisted suicide proponents to the genuine self-determination of people with terminal illnesses."

What these articles convey strongly is that supporters of assisted suicide simply do not care how much collateral damage their campaign for "dying with dignity" will do to people who have lived with their disability for years. Ms Coleman savagely comments: "Proponents of legalized assisted suicide are willing to treat lives ended through abuses of the practice as 'acceptable losses' when balanced against their wish for a pleasant way out and their unwillingness to accept disability, or responsibility for their own suicide."

Third, the danger is not mandated euthanasia, as in Nazi Germany. Rather, it is a subtle and widespread expectation that death is better than disability. "If the legalization of assisted suicide continues, I believe the rank and file will someday see nothing wrong with hastening the deaths of many people," writes Dr Carol J. Gill, director of the Chicago Center for Disability Research. "They will stand by and do nothing to stop it and will endorse the policies and institutions that advance it – not because they are evil people but because it will no longer be evil in our culture to do so. It will be compassionate, respectful, routine."

Fourth, several authors argue forcefully that Oregon's Death with Dignity Act, which is the model for assisted suicide in the US, is deeply flawed. After about 15 years, several intractable problems have emerged. The authors claim that there is very little patient control; that statistics are incomplete; that oversight is minimal and secretive; that safeguards are easily circumvented; and that negligent doctors cannot be prosecuted. Allegations that in Oregon and in the neighbouring state of Washington, which has also legalised assisted suicide, the circumstances of deaths are routinely falsified are especially disturbing. In fact, Washington actually requires that doctors falsify the death certificate by listing the terminal disease as the cause of death rather than the lethal dose of barbiturates.

Nearly always the debate over assisted suicide focuses on disabled people who want to choose death. Why not ask disabled people who want to choose life? They are the biggest stakeholders. Like most academic publications, the *Disability and Health Journal* normally offers obscure and specialised reading. But this month's issue is a must-read for anyone interested in the future of "death with dignity".

Six lessons from death in Belgium

MercatorNet, 4 January 2013

The world was shocked when Belgian doctors euthanized deaf twins who could not bear to be separated.

They look at you with mild detachment. Not aggressive. Not friendly. Not happy. Not sad. Just detached. Two balding middle-aged Belgians with shaved heads, scruffy designer beards, and dark-rimmed oval glasses. The left ear of the man on the right juts out at a sharper angle. But otherwise the two faces are one face. It is the face of 45-year-old identical twins Marc and Eddy Verbessem.

Two weeks before Christmas, a doctor euthanized them at Brussels University Hospital. It was a perfectly legal procedure. All the boxes had been ticked and all the documents signed. The two men were deaf and slowly going blind as well. They had nothing to live for. They qualified.

But nearly everyone felt that there was something inhumanly cold about a society which failed these simple men when they could see and killed them when they couldn't.

As a paradigm case of Belgian euthanasia, it pays to examine how it unfolded and what it reveals about a legalized right to die.

* * * * *

Marc and Eddy Verbessem were born deaf. They never married and they lived together, working as cobblers. When they discovered that they had another congenital disorder, a form of glaucoma, they asked for euthanasia. They could not bear the thought of never seeing each other again.

According to their local doctor, David Dufour, they had other medical problems as well, including debilitating back pain. "All that together made life unbearable," he told the London Telegraph.

Their family opposed their decision. So did the local hospital. It took them nearly two years to find a doctor who was willing to administer a lethal injection under Belgium's euthanasia law. This was Professor Wim Distelmans, a well-known euthanasia activist. He seems proud to have played a key role in "the first time in the world that a 'double euthanasia' has been performed on brothers".

On December 14, dressed in new suits and shoes, reluctantly accompanied by their brother and their parents, they arrived for their appointment with Professor Distelmans. Dr Dufour described their final moments to the media: "They were very happy. It was a relief to see the end of their suffering. They had a cup of coffee in the hall, it went well and [they had] a rich conversation. The separation from their parents and brother was very serene and beautiful. At the last there was a little wave of their hands and then they were gone."

But a fig leaf of smarmy words cannot hide the fact that the twins were killed by their own doctor. Even supporters of euthanasia felt uneasy.

Lesson one: the expanding circle. Under Belgian law euthanasia is allowed if "the patient is in a medically futile condition of constant and unbearable physical or mental suffering that cannot be alleviated, resulting from a serious and incurable disorder caused by illness or accident".

But the Verbessem brothers were not terminally ill. A doctor at their local hospital said, "I do not think this was what the legislation meant by 'unbearable suffering'". Professor Distelmans was nonchalant: "One doctor will evaluate differently than the other."

In an email interview, Jacqueline Herremans, president of Belgium's Association for the Right to Die with Dignity, told me that euthanasia should be made available to many more people:

> When we opened the debate almost 15 years ago, the first thought was for people suffering from incurable cancers. And it is still cancer which is the origin of almost 80% of the cases of euthanasia. But we must admit that suffering may exist in other circumstances. MS, ALS, Parkinson's are obvious. But what about psychiatric disorders without any possibility of cure? What about ageing persons with several medical affections losing their autonomy and seeing no more sense to their life, knowing that tomorrow is going to be worse than today? What about Alzheimer's patients?

Lesson two: euthanasia-minded doctors prefer easy deaths to complicated social work. Marc and Eddy Verbessem's problems were complex. They were shy and withdrawn. Soon they would be not only deaf but deaf and blind. It was difficult for doctors to communicate with them. The easiest way to unravel their social problems was to end them forever.

However, as deaf communities pointed out, being deaf and blind is not a death sentence. After all, America's best-known deafblind person, Helen Keller, travelled the world, wrote books and became an ardent propagandist for socialism.

In fact, a Canadian deafblind activist was dumbfounded. "I wonder if the deafblind Verbessem twins know… the education that was available, the Deafblind community in Belgium around them, the tools that were out there for them to keenly acquire so that their fears of going blind would be soothed with their own amazement and comfort?" Coco Roschaert wrote on her blog.

More to the point: did the doctors who euthanized them know? Did they care?

Lesson three: safeguards are meant to be hurdled. Supporters of legalised euthanasia insist that safeguards in the legislation restrict euthanasia to the most difficult cases. In fact, it is becoming easier and easier to be euthanized in Belgium. A report published late last year by the Brussels-based European Institute of Bioethics has claimed that euthanasia is being "trivialized" and that the law is being monitored by a toothless watchdog. After 10 years of legalised euthanasia and about 5,500 cases, not one case had ever been referred to the police.

The case of the Verbessem twins also shows that procedure is far from transparent. If a prisoner dies in jail, all the facts are made available to the public. If a patient is euthanized, the public may never even find out that it happened. For example, little is known about the health of the twins, how they communicated with the doctors who killed them, whether their social support was adequate, why another hospital had turned down their request, how much counselling they had received.

Doctors naively – or is it arrogantly? – want the public to know as little as possible. "I have been very surprised [that] there is so much interest and debate about this," Dr Dufour said.

Lesson four: if you're disabled, you're in trouble. Professor Chris Gastmans, of the Catholic University of Leuven, criticised the deaths as an impoverished response to disability. "Is this the only humane response that we can offer in such situations? I feel uncomfortable here as ethicist. Today it seems that euthanasia is the only right way to end life. And I think that's not a good thing.

In a society as wealthy as ours, we must find another, caring way to deal with human frailty."

Lesson five: compassionate euthanasia has a price tag. Both Eddy and Marc were charged 180 Euros each for transporting their bodies back home. This macabre detail shouldn't surprise us. China also charges the families of the people it executes. It's called a bullet fee.

Lesson six: not enough Belgians are being euthanized but the government has a plan. In 2011, the last year for which official figures are available, 1133 people were euthanized in Belgium. A few days after the Verbessem brothers died, the government announced that it would amend the law to allow minors and people with dementia to be euthanized as well.

Life? I'm not really that into it any more
MercatorNet, 23 June 2015

Healthy 24-year-old Belgian woman asks for euthanasia.

News flash from Brussels, the nihilism capital of the world! A 24-year-old healthy woman named Laura will soon be euthanized. The reason? *Leven, dat is niets voor mij,* she says: life, that's not for me.

And Belgian doctors are happy to accommodate her, even though she is young and even though she is healthy. If she's not really into life, why not check out the alternative?

A profile in the Belgian newspaper De Morgen tries to explain why Laura has scheduled her death.

She grew up in a dysfunctional household. Her father was drunk and abusive and her mother left him when she was only a year old. From then on she shuttled between her loving grandparents and her mother, who was drunk and slatternly.

By the age of six she was already thinking of suicide. She told the newspaper:

> That thought was very conscious in kindergarten. I was sitting there at the time and I thought, what am I doing here? Or as I was leaving my grandfather for school I thought, 'I don't want to be walking here; I don't want to live at all.'

(She's lucky to be 24 years old. Last year Belgium removed the age limit for euthanasia so that children can ask for it. If it had been legal when she was a toddler, she might not have celebrated her seventh birthday.)

In high school Laura started to self-mutilate and cut her arms. She clearly had serious psychological problems and has ended up in a mental hospital. But at the same time, she has studied acting and set up a comfortable flat. She had ample opportunity to commit suicide, but she never did.

But after years of fighting depression, she has had enough. She wants to jump ship. A date has been set for a lethal injection in her apartment. She has planned her funeral, written songs and drafted a booklet. She insists that the Greg Caswell song "Comes and Goes (in Waves)" should be played.

Isn't anyone going to stop Laura?

Nope.

Three psychiatrists have approved her application for euthanasia. One of them is Lieve Thienpont, a psychiatrist who has just written a book defending euthanasia for people who are suffering psychologically, *Libera Me*. (The Latin words of the book's title are taken from a Catholic prayer for the dead.) Laura went to the book launch recently.

The attitude among the Belgian euthanasia fraternity is that life and death are really not such a big deal. In a powerful feature in *The New Yorker* recently, some of the doctors explained their attitude.

Dr Wim Distelmans, who both does euthanasia and is the chairman of the Federal Control and Evaluation Commission, which reviews euthanasia paperwork to check that doctors observe regulations, said: "If you ask for euthanasia because you are alone, and you are alone because you don't have family to take care of you, we cannot create family."

In other words, people who live in a crumbling social network are on their own. Belgian doctors will do their best to kill them, but not to find a solution to their loneliness.

Another doctor, Dirk De Wachter, a professor of psychiatry at the University of Leuven, told The New Yorker about one of his cases:

> He recently approved the euthanasia of a twenty-five-year-old woman with borderline personality disorder who did not "suffer from depression in the psychiatric sense of the word," he said. "It was more existential; it was impossible for her to have a goal in this life." He said that her parents "came to my office, got on their knees, and begged me, 'Please, help our daughter to die.'"

The law is a teacher. Belgium's euthanasia law is teaching Belgian parents that death is better than life.

For the euthanasia fraternity, life is no longer a treasure. They have revived the ancient pessimism of the Greek philosopher Epicurus, who is renowned for his maxim: "Death, therefore, the most awful of evils, is nothing to us, seeing that, when we are, death is not come, and, when death is come, we are not."

Which is precisely what Etienne Vermeersch, the former president of the Belgian Advisory Committee on Bioethics, and reputedly the most influential intellectual in Flanders (the Dutch-speaking region of Belgium), told *The New Yorker's* reporter: "How can you be afraid of nothing? Nothing can do you no harm ... After death, your relationships are finished. You are in the state you were before conception."

Laura's story suggests that this nihilism among Belgian doctors has affected their willingness to go the extra mile for their patients. She told De Morgen:

> At one stage, my crisis was so severe that it was too much even for the staff. Sometimes I was not allowed in the institute for a few weeks just so they could have a breather. I still find that

incomprehensible, and I don't think highly of psychiatry. I had to save myself but this caused a significant breach of trust.

Whether this is a sign of incompetence or indifference, it still suggests that Belgium's psychiatric services are deficient. It's reminiscent of Belloc's savage verses:

> *Physicians of the Utmost Fame*
> *Were called at once; but when they came*
> *They answered, as they took their Fees,*
> *There is no Cure for this Disease.*

But ultimately the problem is that Belgians have turned the idea of limitless freedom into a national philosophy of nihilism. It is a country where you can define yourself as gay or you can define yourself as straight. You can define yourself as male or you can define yourself as female. And you can define yourself as living or you can define yourself as dead.

Part 2
Dicing with human dignity

The great human dignity heist

It's easy to assert piously that all of us have human dignity; it seems intuitively true. But it's much harder to prove it. The word "dignity" can be interpreted in many different ways, depending on what philosophy you subscribe to. And, in fact, it is a relatively recent concept, dating back to the German Enlightenment philosopher Immanuel Kant. Before then, it was believed that man had been created in the image and likeness of God. But when the very existence of God was challenged, on what foundation could arguments for human dignity be built?

Rationality is the obvious choice. Man is the only animal who can reason, and therefore the only one who can do crosswords, tell jokes, or sing love songs. But rationality itself is in crisis. Some philosophers deny that it is unique to man; others assert that we are moved by our emotions and instincts, not our intellect. In this climate, the notion of human dignity is constantly under attack. This has real life consequences. Behaviour which was once regarded as unworthy of a human being is defended as a legitimate choice. These essays illustrate some of the conundrums which face those of us who believe that human beings are special.

Moral mayhem of murder on the menu

Herald Sun, 15 January 2004

What are the ethics of voluntary cannibalism?

March 9, 2001, was the ultimate bad Herr day for Bernd-Juergen Brandes, a 43-year-old Berlin computer engineer. In the morning he made his will, leaving everything to his gay live-in partner. Then he took a 300km train trip to the central German town of Rotenburg. There he met Armin Meiwes, a mild-mannered 42-year-old computer technician. What they had on their minds was dinner, Meiwes's dinner, to be precise.

Brandes was responding to his request in an internet chat room for a "young well-built man who wants to be eaten". He was willing and Meiwes was ready, with a DIY abattoir and a well-stocked kitchen.

Brandes swallowed 20 sleeping tablets and half a bottle of schnapps. Then Meiwes cut off part of his body and fried it as a snack for them both.

Brandes was bleeding to death, but still not dead when Meiwes stabbed him in the neck after a goodbye kiss. Then Meiwes butchered him and froze the flesh. Eventually he ate about 20kg, washing it down with a South African red. Eventually the police came knocking and he is now being tried in a German court.

The facts are mostly beyond dispute -- Meiwes has cheerfully and remorselessly admitted everything. He had even videotaped the evening's proceedings.

After Hannibal Lecter, reports of real cannibalism seem

banal. There's no pursuit, no suspense, no glamour. Only a bit of deadpan humour. When Brandes learned that both he and Meiwes were both smokers, he apparently said, "Good, smoked meat lasts longer".

The real interest of this case is not that stomach-churning evening, but in this month's courtroom drama. Is cannibalism wrong between consenting adults? Does consent create morality? *Guess Who's Coming for Abendessen* would make a great David Williamson play.

Meiwes cannot be charged with cannibalism, as no German law forbids it. Instead he's been charged with disturbing the peace of the dead, which makes him sound like a neighbour with a blaring stereo.

And it will be difficult to convict Meiwes of murder since Brandes wanted, even pleaded, to be killed and eaten. He will probably be jailed for killing upon request, which makes him sound like voluntary euthanasia advocate Dr Philip Nitschke. This crime is punishable by a mere six months to five years in prison.

German authorities would like to convict Meiwes of murder, but they can only do this if Brandes was mad. But Brandes was a successful professional man who was fully aware of what he was doing. He was an odd bod, admittedly, but most odd bods are technically sane.

In any case, German investigators say there are hundreds of people interested in cannibalism in Europe. Many of them are middle-class professionals. Meiwes even found at least two other volunteers who went as far as having choice cuts marked out on their naked bodies before they called it quits. They can't all be mad.

What the horrific Meiwes-Brandes relationship shows is that

informed consent alone cannot protect human rights. There will always be people who consent to acts that degrade and dehumanise.

It is hard to believe that some citizens, like Bernd-Juergen Brandes, prefer sub-human forms of slavery to freedom. But such people exist. So even if they don't value their own rights and dignity, they need laws to protect them from evil predators like Arwin Meiwes.

This is true for major social issues like prostitution, pornography, deviant sex, drug abuse and gambling. And it is truest of all with "voluntary" euthanasia. However you fence euthanasia with restrictions that guarantee that people who are tired of life will only be killed if they give "informed consent", there will always be monsters who push those fences over.

And who knows what is going on in the mind of the mild-mannered doctor who volunteers to give your ailing mother a lethal injection?

Treat your goldfish well – or else!

MercatorNet, 2 May 2008

Depriving a goldfish of fishy companions has become a crime in Switzerland.

Switzerland is well on its way to becoming the most dignified country in the world, after its federal parliament decreed that goldfish must be protected against physical and psychological abuse. From September 1, Swiss aquariums must have an opaque side to allow the fish live in a natural cycle of day and night. The new law sets rigorous standards for the treatment of all "social animals". It will be an offence, for instance, to keep only one guinea pig or budgerigar. Or one rhinoceros, apparently, because the law also covers pet rhinoceroses.

The Swiss are amongst the best educated people in the world, but they are about to be educated even further. Prospective dog owners will have to pay for and complete a two-part course on the theory and practice of dog ownership. Anglers will also be required to take a course on handling fish with dignity.

The Swiss are pioneers in this field. In 1992 Switzerland was the first country in the world to begin to phase out battery hens. Since then the law has become even tougher. In 2006, for instance, a researcher was forbidden to give thirsty monkeys a drink of water because a reward mechanism to get them to carry out a task was deemed harmful to their dignity.

And if that is not absurd enough, it now seems possible that the ever-expanding boundaries of non-human dignity will include plants.

Dicing with human dignity

The Swiss Constitution requires respect for "the dignity of creation when handling animals, plants and other organisms". The body in charge of interpreting this Delphic phrase, the Federal Ethics Committee on Non-Human Biotechnology, has just released a discussion paper about the dignity of plants. In due course its astonishing conclusions could become law.

Amongst them is that "decapitation of wild flowers at the roadside without rational reason" is essentially a crime. In fact, the committee was unanimous in its agreement that any "arbitrary harm caused to plants[is] morally impermissible." Genetic modification of plants would be permitted -- but only if their "independence", including their reproductive ability, is ensured. This could mean, for instance, that producing sterile roses or seedless fruit would become an offence under Swiss law.

None of this is a joke. The world's leading science journal, *Nature*, recently reported that Swiss biologists are worried. Funding for their work might get cut off if they offend the dignity of plants.

Switzerland's passion for the dignity of all creatures great and small, however, rings hollow in view of its treatment of human beings. It is one of the few countries in the world where assisted suicide is legal. The best-known agency for DIY euthanasia, a Zurich-based group called – what else? – Dignitas, recently opened its thanatorium near Switzerland's biggest legal brothel. Surely that violates one of the numerous provisions in the constitution guaranteeing human dignity. As it is now, there seems to be about as much bureaucracy involved in killing a Swiss goldfish as there is in killing a human being. (Special chemicals are required since flushing fish down the toilet has been deemed undignified.)

The poor, befuddled Swiss have clearly lost the plot on what dignity is and who is entitled to it.

But they are not alone. Around the world the concept of human dignity is in crisis. Influential government reports in country after country are now condescendingly placing scare quotes on either side of the phrase "human dignity".

Britain's Human Fertilisation and Embryology Authority last year complained that "it is difficult to gain a consensus on the definition of human dignity". And the Irish Council on Bioethics last month declared that "its exact meaning is elusive". The President's Council on Bioethics in the US has just released a fat report which tries to clarify what it is. Although many of the contributors defend it, neuroscientist Patricia Churchland guts "human dignity" of all content. She contends, like many of her colleagues, that morality and free will are essentially illusory and that past defenders of "human dignity" have been self-righteous, totalitarian fanatics.

The trigger for this controversy is a widely-discussed paper written four years ago by an American bioethicist, Ruth Macklin, in the British Medical Journal. She stated bluntly that "dignity is a useless concept in medical ethics and can be eliminated without any loss of content."

Well, the Swiss folderol suggests we will all be very sorry when "human dignity" is eliminated. As the scope of human dignity in Switzerland has shrunk to the point that international death tourism there has become a boutique business, the scope of non-human dignity has expanded. This is to be expected. For years the radical fringe of animal rights activists has defended animals against violence by using violence against humans.

What is unexpected is that there seems to be no brake on the ever-expanding circle of dignity. You would think that it must stop somewhere above spiders and slugs. But the Swiss experience suggests otherwise. Once the DNA of human dignity has been tampered with, it keeps expanding by some crazy logic, unrestrained by common sense, until it includes plants, and even "other organisms". It is already burdening Swiss farmers with additional costs and hampering the work of Swiss scientists. Now it threatens to turn treading on wildflowers into a crime. And it might not stop there. What constitutes respect for the dignity of bacteria and viruses must send shivers through the Swiss pharmaceutical industry.

The Swiss need to recover the conviction that human beings deserve a special status because they are unique in the universe, the only beings with reason and free will. That is not only the wellspring of our dignity, but the source of our obligation to treat animals and plants with due care. Otherwise they will end up conferring rights upon irrational beings who cannot appreciate their dignity by stealing them from rational beings who can.

Human dignity, what a stupid idea!

MercatorNet, 17 May 2008

At least, that's what a psychology professor at Harvard thinks.

In the minds of most people, human dignity is a cornerstone of bioethics. After all, bioethics was partly inspired by horrific abuses of human dignity by Nazi doctors. To protect it, the new United Nations ratified in 1948 the Universal Declaration of Human Rights. This recognised "the inherent dignity and... the equal and inalienable rights of all members of the human family". And nearly 40 national constitutions ratified since World War II have referred explicitly to human dignity. Like life, liberty and the pursuit of happiness, human dignity is one of those notions that is in the air we breathe.

But not, it turns out, the air breathed by professional bioethicists. In fact, low-intensity academic warfare is sputtering along over a 2003 proposal by Ruth Macklin, at Albert Einstein College of Medicine in New York, that "human dignity" (scare quotes essential) should be junked. This doesn't mean that she wanted to ill-treat people. Rather, she regarded the two words as highfalutin baggage smuggled in from religion which can and should be discarded. They were either too vague to be meaningful or they simply restated other notions, such as respect for autonomy or capacity for rational thought.

The controversy provoked the President's Council for Bioethics, a government study group set up by President Bush, to respond with a fat book of essays which, for the most part, defend the disputed notion. And this in turn provoked Steven

Pinker to rebut it in the most influential opinion journal in the US, *The New Republic*, under the inflammatory headline, "The Stupidity of Dignity".

If you haven't heard of Steven Pinker, you obviously don't read the *New York Times* much. He is one of America's top public intellectuals, with a number of best-selling books on how the mind and language work to his credit. Back in 2004 *Time* magazine called him one of the 100 most influential people in the world. He is also a professor of evolutionary psychology at Harvard University, which gives his theory even more weight. And this theory, repeated over and over in his writings, is that "the mind is what the brain does". This is more or less the theme of his book, *How the Mind Works*. It is an increasing popular view among neuroscientists.

Surprisingly for a distinguished academic, most of what Pinker had to say was more or less personal abuse. He attacked the Council as a body stacked with Catholic "theocons" and led by a conservative Jew, Leon Kass, whom he calls "pro-death" and "anti-freedom". It all sounded a bit like Rush Limbaugh on Hillary Clinton. But I admit that I became seriously disturbed when Pinker quoted Kass's severe condemnation of the practice of licking ice cream cones in public places as inconsistent with human dignity. No way José. Triple-scoop peppermint-and-chocolate-chip ice creams are not something I am going to give up, even for the sake of human dignity.

Thankfully, though, I took a deep breath and read on. Dr Kass is the author of numerous books and his views on ice cream must have come from one of them, but they did not appear in the Council's collection of essays. Pinker had been beating America's leading defender of "human dignity" over the head with a red herring, which is even more undignified than slurping in public.

No doubt there is a personal element in this dust-up. This is not the first clash between the two scholars. Writing in the journal *Commentary* last year, Kass's defence of a non-materialist account of human nature against the Harvard academic was scathing: "One hardly knows which is the more impressive, the height of Pinker's arrogance or the depth of his shallowness... he does not understand that the empowering organization of materials -- the vital form -- is not itself material." Perhaps Pinker was still feeling the sting of the lash.

Eventually, however, Pinker's spleen dribbled away and he came to grips with "human dignity" itself. He criticised it for being relative (some people find public consumption of ice cream dignified), fungible (colonoscopies are undignified and we willing endure them), and harmful (think of Saddam Hussein's highly dignified military parades). Human dignity, it seems, is a nasty business. It puts us at risk of being arrested by "the ice cream police" for perfectly acceptable things like therapeutic cloning. Why rabbit on about the "squishy, subjective notion" of dignity when you can jog along perfectly well with clear, sharp-edged ideas like autonomy and respect for persons?

Come again?

While "human dignity" is an idea which certainly requires extensive clarification and precise definition, "respect for persons" and "autonomy" are as squishy as a wet sponge. I would have thought that a Harvard prof would be more discerning. For instance, are dolphins or chimpanzees "persons", too? Should Japanese fishermen be jailed for violating the person rights of minke whales? And is a sleeping person autonomous? A comatose person? A two-day-old infant?

Along with human dignity, Pinker seems to have jettisoned 2,500 years of non-materialist Western philosophy. Man, *homo sapiens*, is an animal, but in the words of Aristotle, he is a rational animal. Any analysis of man which fails to take into account his evident non-material capacity for beauty, or abstraction, or dreams of the future will inevitably put human dignity between scare quotes. Pinker, astonishingly, is virtually blind to philosophical discourse. This explains why he zeroes in on Kass's scandalous opinions on ice cream cones and ignores his defence of man's capacity for "reason, freedom, judgment, and moral concern". Dialoguing with Pinker about human dignity is rather like discussing the chemistry of H2O with someone who doesn't believe in oxygen.

When I began to read Pinker's article, I was filled with foreboding about the future of bioethics. But by the end, I realized that it was far from bad news. If the best way to construct a philosophical defence of therapeutic cloning, for instance, is to throw "human dignity" overboard, people will think twice about it. While ridiculing human dignity may raise a few chuckles in the Harvard Faculty Club, it will never play in Peoria. Denigrating human dignity is a brain wave without a future.

Plastinated People

Australasian Science, May 2010

Exhibits of human remains in garish poses raise issues of human dignity.

Human dignity is a motherhood concept like freedom of speech or the brotherhood of man. But what happens when it conflicts with the motherhood concept of autonomy —the ability to make free and independent decisions? An example of this dilemma is dwarf-tossing. When a town in France banned it in 2002, one of the dwarfs objected. He was participating freely, and being treated as a basketball was his livelihood.

The case went all the way to the Conseil d'État, the French counterpart to our High Court, which dismissed the dwarf's appeal to autonomy. Allowing himself to be used as a mere projectile compromised his dignity, it said. The dwarf then appealed to the United Nations' Human Rights and Anti-Discrimination Committee, which upheld the ban "in order to protect public order and considerations of human dignity".

Calibrating the balance between autonomy and human dignity is so tricky that some bioethicists have taken to denying the existence of human dignity altogether. A few years ago, for instance, Ruth Macklin was widely applauded by many of her colleagues when she wrote in the *British Medical Journal* that human dignity was a "useless concept" compared with autonomy. "Human dignity" meant different things to different people, she wrote, and since she couldn't find a rigorously logical definition she said it should be scrapped.

Granted, autonomy is important, but there's something scary

about bioethics without human dignity. After all, it was revulsion at the atrocities committed by Nazi doctors in the death camps that gave rise to modern bioethics. Surely something more than a violation of the victims' autonomy was involved.

For instance, how should we evaluate modern exhibits of plastinated bodies? Plastination is a technique used by anatomists to preserve specimens for students but, like many useful technologies, it can be used for dubious purposes. A German anatomist, Gunther von Hagens, has turned plastination into a money-spinner. Since 1995 his flayed and partially dissected corpses – a man playing chess with his brain exposed, a man striding a rearing horse, a woman and her baby in the eighth month of pregnancy and so on – have been touring the world. You can see the muscles, tendons, bones and organs bulge and stretch. A recent exhibit in Berlin featured a copulating couple.

"These are blockbuster shows," according to an American analyst of the museum exhibition business. "We haven't seen anything like this since the robotic dinosaurs in the 1980s."

Why do the crowds like them? It's a mixture of curiosity and disgust. The exhibits do teach a bit of anatomy, but the sight of plastinated genitalia must surely be part of the attraction for the millions.

So is there anything unethical about these exhibits?

Bioethicists like Macklin would say not if the people had agreed to donate their bodies, but even on this score the exhibits might be unethical. Von Hagens and his competitors have been dogged by allegations that some of the bodies, at least, belong to executed criminals from China, Kyrgyzstan or elsewhere. When an exhibit toured England recently, *The Lancet* harrumphed that its paperwork was dodgy. "Assurance that all remains on public display were donated with informed consent of the deceased, is imperative," it said in an editorial.

But what if all the "i"s were jotted and the "t"s were crossed? After all, thousands of people have agreed to donate their bodies. "It's something that you want to do instead of being ashes or worm food – to be some kind of asset instead of being in the ground," one woman said. Von Hagens has even claimed that two-thirds of the males who donated their bodies to his company and one-third of the females agreed to the use of their bodies for the representation of sexual acts.

But isn't there something deeply unsettling about all this that an informed consent form cannot put to rest? These exhibits had been living, breathing people. Isn't undressing them, treating them as commercial property and displaying them in poses designed to elicit ribald smirks a degradation of the very idea of embodied humanity?

If they did consent, did their loved ones consent? Is the human body just an artefact? What lessons does an exhibit impart to children about the meaning of human existence and the existence of human dignity?

Even the patron saint of "autonomy", the 19th century British philosopher John Stuart Mill, put a limit to autonomy. A contract to sell oneself into slavery, he said, would be "null and void". Certainly our gut feelings about human dignity have to be more rigorously expressed, but it would be a tragedy for bioethics if the idea was scrapped.

The French courts got it right. There are some things that autonomy cannot justify.

Tears for Middle Pleistocene human Cranium 14
MercatorNet, 6 April 2009

An amazing archaeological finding in Spain reveals the deep humanity of our distant ancestors.

There is a poignant, passionate poem by the Australian poet A.D. Hope about a thousand-year-old bone inscribed with Viking runes. It concludes:

> And, in a foreign tongue,
> A man, who is not he,
> Reads and his heart is wrung
> This ancient grief to see,
> And thinks: When I am dung,
> What bone shall speak for me?

Perhaps an anthropologist with a poetic bent will be inspired to write something similar after reading the latest issue of the *Proceedings of the National Academy of Sciences*. Hidden under the dry headline of "Craniosynostosis in the Middle Pleistocene human Cranium 14 from the Sima de los Huesos, Atapuerca, Spain" is another tale of ancient grief. So ancient -- 530,000 years ago -- that the thread of humanity linking it to us all but snaps.

Cranium 14 was discovered in the famous archaeological site of Atapuerca. Scattered throughout several caves in the area are the bones and tools of the earliest humans found in Europe. The most interesting findings are to be found in Sima de los Huesos (the pit of the bones). This site is located at the bottom of a 13-metre (50-foot) deep chimney which has to be accessed by scrambling through caves. Twenty-eight people of both sexes rest in pieces, smashed into thousands of fragments.

The great human dignity heist

No one knows exactly how and why the bones tumbled there, but it may have been a burial ground. Another theory is that they were washed down when the cave flooded. No matter. The point is that more than 30 fragments belonged to a little girl aged between 5 and 12. Nameless now, she has been christened Cranium 14 by the anthropologists.

Any relics this old offer precious clues to the lives of our distant ancestors. But when the researchers reconstructed Cranium 14's fragments, they discovered something very surprising: she appears to have been severely mentally retarded. They know this because she clearly suffered from craniosynostosis, a birth defect in which the skull segments close too early, producing facial deformities and interfering with the development of the brain.

The particular skull distortion of the child in Sima de Huesos affects fewer than 6 in 200,000 individuals in living humans. It is distressing for parents. The head can be large and misshapen; the eyes can bulge out. The children can be blind and deaf. Their limbs may be deformed. They may have seizures and feed poorly. Cranio-facial surgery works wonders and after many, many operations, an affected child can lead something like a normal life. Even so, the story of a child with the condition makes for painful reading. Many doctors would advise mothers to terminate the pregnancy.

Here's the remarkable thing. The hunter-gatherer Middle Pleistocene family of Cranium 14 must have cared for the child or she would not have survived for at least five years, and perhaps as many as 12 years. In the dry-as-dust words of the article, "It is obvious that the [Sima de Huesos] hominid species did not act against the abnormal/ill individuals during the infancy, as has happened along our own history many times and in many cultures".

They go on to say: "Cranium 14 is the earliest documented case of craniosynostosis with resulting neurocranial, brain deformities, and, very likely, asymmetries of the facial skeleton. Despite these handicaps, this individual survived for >5 years, suggesting that her/his pathological condition was not an impediment to receive the same attention as any other Middle Pleistocene Homochild".

Were the hunter-gatherer Middle Pleistocene hearts of the family of Cranium 14 wrung with ancient grief when she died? We don't know. We know only that her bones speak of tenderness and compassion. Season after season, under unimaginably harsh conditions, they tended her with callused hands until she died. Nowadays, if her disability had been detected early enough, she would probably be aborted.

Sometimes civilisation is a mixed blessing.

Part 3
War heroes

In a sense, bioethics is the study of the limitations of the human condition. It could the suffering of infertility, of old age, of chronic pain, of being disabled, of caring for the disabled, or death or even our condition as mortals who long for immortality. On a theoretical level, bioethics establishes the limits of what can be done to relieve this suffering. But on an existential level, it only leads us to the threshold of making sense of suffering, of giving it meaning.

If we want meaning, the best place to start is the lives of people who transcend pain. They show that it is possible to be happy in the midst of discomfort, disability, pain and dying. What is their secret?

Seeking respect for human life

Herald Sun, 21 May 2002

Austrians have given a final resting place to the remains of voiceless and defenceless children murdered by the Nazi doctors as part of their research.

In Vienna's central cemetery 789 children tortured and murdered by Nazi doctors were laid to rest last month. Two black urns with the brains of two of them were given a formal public burial. The remains of about 600 other children were buried privately over a two-week period.

These physically or mentally handicapped children died between 1940 and 1945. They had been sent to a prestigious hospital, Am Spiegelgrund, for quality treatment. Instead, their "worthless lives" were poisoned with sleeping tablets and starved until they died of pneumonia.

In life the Nazis regarded them as "useless eaters", but in death they were far from useless to the doctor who killed them. For decades, their brains, carefully preserved in formaldehyde or dissected for anatomical slides, were used for neurological research.

The doctor, Heinrich Gross, escaped justice after the War and went on to become a leading neurologist. He wrote psychiatric reports for Austrian courts until 1998 and published many papers on brain deformations, basing his work mainly on his Spiegelgrund victims. In 1975, Gross was even awarded a medal of honour for his scientific contributions.

Atrocities like these have made Austrians and Germans

wary of human embryo experimentation. Victims of the Nazi ideology know all too well that respect for human life is a fragile virtue. And before Parliament ratifies the decision of the Council of Australian Government to allow destructive research on unwanted IVF embryos, we ought to reflect on the lessons of Dr Gross's victims.

Don't get me wrong. Embryo research is NOT Nazi-inspired.

This would be a gross distortion of largely well-intentioned efforts to cure children and adults suffering from degenerative diseases.

More to the point, Nazism was an archaic form of eugenic socialism. With the gigantic power of the Nazi state behind them, German and Austrian doctors implemented this, betraying their commitment to protect and heal the weakest and most defenceless members of society, the mentally and physically disabled.

Destructive human embryo research, on the other hand, is largely a profit-driven, free-market affair which meshes neatly with the privatisation and outsourcing of eugenics. An eminent UK psychologist, Richard Lynn, has even just published a book, *Eugenics: A Reassessment*, arguing that it's time for a fresh look at the unjustly maligned practice engineering the genetic quality of the population. It fits nicely into our consumer mentality, he says.

No, destructive embryo research is not Nazi-inspired, but you would have to be Blind Freddy to overlook the parallels.

In 1949, the chief medical consultant to the prosecution at the Nuremberg War Crimes Tribunal, Dr Leo Alexander, reflected on the dangers of unravelling the thread of respect for human life: "it is important to realise that the infinitely small wedged-in lever from which this entire trend of mind received its impetus was the attitude toward the non-rehabilitable sick."

In the 21st Century, the impetus is the fact that because embryos are "unwanted" or "surplus" or going to die anyway, they are unworthy of the incipient life they do have.

The good intentions of skilful doctors do not weaken the parallel. Nazi doctors at Nuremberg made constant allusions to medical ethics and the Hippocratic oath in their testimony. They even seem to have convinced themselves that their crimes were consistent with their high principles.

To be sure, IVF embryos do not look like grown-up persons. But they do look like one-minute old persons. They are self-directed, purposeful bundles of potential babyhood, childhood and adulthood. However, like the murdered Austrian children, they are voiceless and defenceless. To the ideologues of the consumer society, just as to Heinrich Gross, they are valueless lives with invaluable body parts.

And tragically, judging from the current record of progress, the dissection of unwanted IVF embryos may not be value for money. Thus far, not a single patient has ever been treated successfully with human embryonic stem cells. Not one.

On the other hand, adult stem cells, extracted from placentas, children or adults without the slightest ethical complication, have already treated patients successfully for a number of conditions, including Parkinson's disease, Alzheimer's disease and diabetes.

The Austrians have given us a way to cope with the thousands of parentless embryos in the freezers of IVF clinics. We, too, can bury them.

Let's repudiate the callous consumerism of "use it or lose it".

Dame Cicely Saunders

MercatorNet, 30 July 2005

The remarkable woman who founded the modern hospice movement died this month in the institution she founded.

Dame Cicely Saunders ~ 22 June 1918 - 14 July 2005

Everyone knows of Florence Nightingale, the nurse whose selflessness and energy in caring for soldiers during the Crimean War transformed hospitals and made nursing a true profession. Her contemporary counterpart was another Briton, Dame Cicely Saunders, who died earlier this month at the age of 87. It was the capstone of a lifetime specialising in care for the dying.

Dame Cicely's achievement was to begin the modern hospice movement in 1967. There are now hundreds of hospices for the dying in Britain and in more than 95 countries around the world. Without her work, the euthanasia movement would undoubtedly have been far more persuasive and legalised euthanasia would have spread much further. She showed that it was possible to die peacefully and without great pain. For her, dying was not something to be feared but was "as natural as being born". Partly due to her influence, palliative care has become recognised as a distinct medical speciality.

Dame Cicely was a woman of wisdom. Although she was an eminent clinician and researcher, she knew that care for the dying was not simply a matter of managing patients' pain. She developed a theory of "total pain" which included its emotional, social, and spiritual elements. "The whole experience for a patient includes anxiety, depression, and fear; concern for the family who will become bereaved; and often a need to find some meaning in the situation, some deeper reality in which to trust," she said.

Dame Cicely was also a woman with deeply Christian convictions, but her hospices were open to people of all persuasions, and to those who had none. "I once asked a man who knew he was dying what he needed above all in those who were caring for him," she once said. "He said, 'For someone to look as if they are trying to understand me.' Indeed it is impossible to understand fully another person, but I never forgot that he did not ask for success but only that someone should care enough to try."

That wisdom was hard-won. Her well-to-do father disapproved of her interest in nursing and so she enrolled at Oxford instead. When World War II broke out, however, she took up nursing. But her back gave her trouble and she had to switch to a degree in social work. In 1945 her parents divorced and she converted from agnosticism to evangelical Christianity. This happened all of a sudden, during a holiday in Cornwall with some Christian friends. "It was as though I suddenly felt the wind behind me rather than in my face," she later said. "I thought to myself: please let this be real. I prayed to know how best to serve God."

The answer came the next year when she fell in love with a dying Polish Jew named David Tasma, the first of three romantic attachments to Polish men. "He needed to make his peace with the God of his fathers, and the time to sort out who he was," she recalled. "We discussed the idea of somewhere that could have helped him do this better than a busy hospital ward." When Tasma died, he bequeathed Saunders £500 -- no mean sum in those days -- to start a hospice. "I'll be a window in your home," he said.

Her mission in life was now clear to her: founding a home

where the dying would receive the best medical care along with affection and understanding. A doctor told her that people would not listen to a nurse, so at the age of 33 she began a medical degree. In 1957 she qualified and obtained a research scholarship in pain management for the incurably ill, at the same time working in a hospice for the dying poor run by Catholic Sisters of Charity.

There she met the second Pole in her life, Antoni Michniewicz, who showed her what death could be like when it was surrounded by loving care. He inspired her to name her own hospice for people in the final stage of life's journey after Saint Christopher, the patron of travellers.

In 1967 she opened St Christopher's in London. Initially it had 54 in-patient beds with respite care and a home care service. The years of planning which preceded this also brought to light Dame Cicely's other sterling qualities as a medical administrator, a fund-raiser and publicist for her vision.

Three years after the death of Antoni she spotted a picture of the Crucifixion in a gallery which she thought would be appropriate for the hospice. She contacted the Polish artist, Marian Bohusz-Szyszko, and ended up falling in love with him even though he was 18 years older. He was a devout Catholic who still supported his estranged wife and it was only after she died that Cicely married him. She was 61 and he was 79 and in poor health. She gave him constant nursing care and he ended his days in St Christopher's in 1995.

She never gave up working, although she retired from active involvement in St Christopher's in 1985. In 2002 she launched the Cicely Saunders Foundation which aims to promote research into palliative care, with a focus on collaboration amongst the different specialties of healthcare.

According to an obituary in the London *Times*, many years ago she told a questioner at a symposium that she would prefer to die with a cancer which would give her time to reflect upon her life and to put her material and spiritual affairs in order. And that is what happened. She passed away at St Christopher's of breast cancer.

As a clinician, Cicely Saunders will probably be remembered for a relatively novel method of pain relief -- administering sedation to achieve a steady state in which a dying patient can still remain conscious and have a reasonable quality of life, instead of reacting to surging pain with intermittent sedation. She opposed euthanasia, arguing that everyone had a right to die well, without pain and with dignity, and that death can be a positive experience.

But on a deeper level, she was able to speak of death as a natural and positive part of a complete life, translating some features of her own Christian approach into a secular idiom.

Those who work in palliative care may have to realise that they, too, are being challenged to face this dimension for themselves. Many, both helper and patient, live in a secularised society and have no religious language. Some will, of course, still be in touch with their religious roots and find a familiar practice, liturgy, or sacrament to help their need. Others, however, will not. For them insensitive suggestions by well-meaning practitioners will be unwelcome.

However, if we can come not only in our professional capacity but in our common, vulnerable humanity there may be no need of words on our part, only of concerned listening. For those who do not wish to share their deepest needs, the way care is given can reach the most hidden places. Feelings of fear and guilt may seem inconsolable, but many of us have sensed that an inner journey has taken place and that a person nearing the end of life has found peace. Important relationships may be developed or reconciled at this time and a new sense of self-worth develop.

The loudest voices in today's debates over euthanasia are often its champions, doctors whose credentials include public defiance of the law by killing depressed and lonely patients. But in the long run, it will probably be the softer and more humane voice of Dame Cicely Saunders who helped hundreds to a peaceful death: "You matter because you are you, and you matter to the last moment of your life."

The last woman in an iron lung
MercatorNet, 6 June 2008

> *An inspirational Tennessee woman who died last week was the last American to live in an iron lung.*

Dianne Odell

Born, 13 February 1947 in Jackson, Tennessee. Died, 28 May 2008 in Jackson, Tennessee.

It used to begin with a stiff neck and a bad headache and fever and weak legs. The worst part was being in hospital away from your parents, who were frantic, of course, because so many kids were paralysed and dying in another polio epidemic. Just about every summer in the 40s and 50s there would be one somewhere. People were scared stiff. Don't drink from public fountains. Avoid swimming pools. Stay away from movie theatres.

And there was no cure.

Oddly enough, the culprit was cleanliness. In backward times babies crawled around in polio-laden dirt and filth. After a brief bout of flu-like symptoms they became immune. But starchy clean 20th century American babies never became infected. And when the disease struck unimmunised children and adults, it struck hard. In 1952, the disease's last hurrah, there were 58,000 cases. About 3,000 died of suffocation when their respiratory muscles became paralysed. About 21,000 ended up with leg braces or wheelchairs after the disease destroyed nerves and left muscles withered and bones stunted.

Then in the late 50s came the Salk and Sabine vaccines and

suddenly it was game over for poliomyelitis, at least in the United States. It became a forgotten disease. You only read the word polio in the newspaper nowadays when it flares up in distant cities overseas with hard-to-remember names -- although in recent years some survivors complain of a mysterious fatigue which doctors call post-polio syndrome.

But for a handful of Americans post-polio syndrome was literally all-encompassing. They had the worst kind, bulbo-spinal, which destroyed the nerves which controlled their breathing. An iron lung had to breathe for them and they ended up spending whole lives inside a gigantic mechanical jelly roll.

Dianne Odell was the last of them.

It was 1950 when Dianne caught polio in Jackson, Tennessee. She was three years old. After an epidemic struck, hospital wards were full of the deafening racket of rattling machines with small children inside. After a few weeks, many polio children started breathing on their own and left. Dianne never did. She lived the rest of her life in her 7-foot, 750-pound "yellow submarine".

"I remember how much my legs hurt and I went to Mama and told her," she wrote in an unfinished autobiography. "I never walked again after that. I screamed from the hot towels they put on my legs. I remember a lot. I asked my daddy, 'Will I have to live in this thing always?'"

At first, the answer was no, not always. Initially, she could spend three hours outside it every day. When she was 13, she used one of her brief escapes to be baptised in her parents' bathtub. But after 20 or so, home was an iron lung in a small house.

The iron lung wheezed and throbbed 24/7. An electric pump regulated the pressure in her chest and forced air in and out of her lungs. Dianne would lie on her back, with her head protruding from one end of the airtight torpedo. She stared overhead at a mirror hanging above her face so that she could peer around her room. Through a window in her room she could see the tops of trees in the yard.

An iron lung is a simple contraption, no more complicated than a washing machine. The main problem is ensuring that the electricity which keeps the pump running never goes off. In 1957, a storm knocked the power out and her family and rescue workers had to pump by hand. It happened again in 1974. Eventually, in 1995, the Tennessee Valley Authority donated a generator which was supposed to kick in automatically if the power failed.

Her parents never thought of institutionalising her. She was their daughter. No one ever mentioned euthanasia. They fed her and cleaned her and monitored the throbbing machine. Over a two-way radio Dianne attended the local high school and even tried to attend Freed-Hardeman University. She never finished, but it gave her an honorary doctorate in psychology anyway. She wrote a children's novel which sold 100,000 copies and tutored children and campaigned over the phone for politicians she supported.

She had a sunny disposition which her disability and constant pain could not crush. "Don't you ever ask, why me?" people would say. And Dianne would answer in her deep Southern drawl, "Why not me? Who am I?" Celebrities came to be photographed with her and to glimpse something of the grandeur of the human spirit. Tennessee's favourite son, the inventor of the internet and a former Vice-President, Al Gore, gave her a kiss.

One of her cherished sayings was "no man is poor who has friends". "If that's true," she used to say, "then I must be the richest woman alive, and bells are ringing all over West Tennessee, for there are many angels among us. When you have faith, family and friends, you have more than enough to get you through any rough times in your life."

She needed those friends. Her family was not wealthy and her parents' health was bad in recent years. Medicare refused to foot the bill for her care because Dianne couldn't tick the boxes next to skilled nursing care, physical therapy, speech therapy or occupational therapy. So the American can-do spirit took over and friends, admirers and the local church organised fund-raisers to support her.

She was the last surviving American to use an iron lung. In the 50s, a positive pressure ventilator was developed which gave other patients more mobility. But Dianne's spine was curved like a gigantic S and she couldn't use it.

Year by year the number of iron lung users in the United States declined. Some switched to the new-fangled technology; others died. Iron lungs were no longer a money-making proposition. One day Dianne received a letter from the owner. It read: "Due to the age of these products, effective no later than March 1, 2004, Respironics Colorado will no longer be able to procure service parts to support or repair these devices." The company gave Dianne her device and somehow loving family and friends found the parts to keep it running. Her life depended on it.

On May 28, at 3am, a thunderstorm knocked out the power to her house. Then the emergency generator failed. Dianne Odell died as her father and brother-in-law took turns pumping the iron lung in which she had lived for 58 years.

One of the famous people in her life, actor David Keith, a fellow Tennesseean, summed up her life: "Dianne was a window through which you could see the way God intended the world to be."

Chevalier in the fight for human dignity
MercatorNet, 2 November 2010

France has just given its highest dignity to a courageous woman who battled locked-in syndrome and quadriplegia to fight for the disabled.

France has just awarded the Légion d'honneur to a woman who beat locked-in syndrome but has been a quadriplegic for 30 years. Fifty-six-year-old Maryannick Pavageau received the distinction for years of battling for the dignity of the handicapped and disabled.

In 1984, when she was 29, she had a stroke which left her completely paralysed. For months she was in a coma. When she awakened, she could only move her eyelids. Later she recovered some speech and a bit of movement in some fingers. But she still required round-the-clock professional care when she returned home after 32 months in hospital. She had a husband and a two-year-old daughter and she could barely communicate with them. It must have been devastating for an active woman working as a lawyer and marriage counsellor.

But Mme Pavageau is a woman of determination and courage. "When I discovered the state I was in, it never occurred to me to ask 'why me?'" she says. "Instead, I said, 'what's next?'"

Despite her gigantic handicaps she raised her daughter Myriam — who is now a diplomat —has travelled as far as Rome and Beijing, and has become an activist for the disabled and against euthanasia. Jean Leonetti, a cardiologist and a deputy in the French parliament who wrote a 2008 report for the government which slammed the door shut on the legalisation of euthanasia, was so impressed with her intelligence and courage that he devoted a chapter in his book on euthanasia to describing how she managed to cope with her disability. Its title was "la force immobile".

Her interview with Dr Leonetti, as he gathered material for his report, is very moving.

> Every painful situation calls for respect but is just saying that enough when people cry for help? We must refine the meaning of words, step back, and not get caught up in waves of emotion. Let us distinguish between what is presented as a gesture of love and what is actually a great cry and desperate quest for love…
>
> The time has certainly come for associations which defend the weak to join the current debate and unequivocally affirm that everyone, regardless of his handicap, his accident, his discouragement, retains a place in society and that there are no limits to human dignity.
>
> I confess that sometimes I feel discouraged. I get completely fed up.
>
> But as a response to our deep discouragement, are we only entitled to what is hypocritically called the ultimate 'act of love'? I fully recognize that our situation can sometimes be difficult. Even if there is relief for physical pain, there is the mental suffering. but you can hang on, you're not alone. We must keep up out hope, if only in the progress of science.

A resident of the town of Sainte Nazaire, on the Atlantic coast, Mme Pavageau gave an interview about her life to the local newspaper after this week's award:

"All life is worth living," she said. "It can be beautiful, regardless of the state we are in. And change is always possible. That is the message of hope that I wish to convey. I am firmly against euthanasia because it is not physical suffering that guides the desire to die but a moment of discouragement, feeling like a burden... All those who ask to die are mostly looking for love."

Despite her paralysis and her need for round-the-clock care, she was inspired by her love for her family to fight for life. "My life is not what it could have been but it's my life. Finally, I have been faithful to my values. I had the love of my husband and my daughter Myriam, who was two years old at the time and that gave me the strength to fight. Despite my difficulties speaking Myriam has always understood me."

Two years ago, she wrote an article in which she strongly criticised discussion of euthanasia in the media. "Public statements produce unexpected collateral damage amongst people suffering from serious illness such as Locked-In Syndrome. We are constant consumers of TV and radio programs. In response to our deep discouragement – and who is free from that? – we are only offered this final right, hypocritically baptised as a sign of love.

"A recent study on the quality of life of locked-in syndrome patients found, to the astonishment of the medical profession, that when asked 'if you had a heart attack, would you want to be resuscitated?', the great majority of us answered: Yes."

She is proud to become a Chevalier of the Legion d'Honneur, France's highest decoration, although she looks upon it as recognition for everyone whose dignity has been diminished by being called a "vegetable". She smiles as she tells the reporter, "If someone had told me that this would happen to me someday, I would never have believed it!"

An African martyr for both science and faith
MercatorNet, 10 September 2015

Benedict Daswa, a South African school teacher, has been declared South Africa's first saint

South Africa will be celebrating a hero of conscience on Sunday – Benedict Daswa, a Catholic school teacher who was murdered in 1990 for opposing witchcraft. A delegate from Pope Francis will beatify him as a martyr in Limpopo, the northeasternmost province.

Daswa, a Catholic convert, was born in 1946. He and his wife Eveline had eight children. He was respected for his community spirit, his hard work and his piety. In 1977 he became principal of a local primary school.

However, he made enemies for opposing traditional witchcraft. In 1976, his local soccer team was on the skids and some of his team mates wanted to consult a sorcerer. Daswa resigned and started his own team.

In late 1989, the local district was hit by heavy rain and lightning. When the storms returned in January 1990, the elders demanded that everyone contribute five Rand to pay for a traditional healer who would identify the witch who had brought the storms.

Daswa spurned this as a superstition. He said that storms were just a natural phenomenon and that he would refuse to pay for a witchdoctor.

On February 2 a mob ambushed him while driving home. He sprinted for safety in a nearby house but he was caught. One of the crowd brained him with a knobkerrie (war club) and boiling water was poured over his head to ensure that he was dead. Before dying Daswa said, "God, into Your hands receive my spirit". Several people were arrested but the case was dismissed for lack of evidence.

Benedict Daswa's life and death pose some fascinating questions.

For starters, why isn't Richard Dawkins presiding at the beatification? Couldn't Daswa be described as a martyr for the Enlightenment, for science? After all, in the last 500 years, the closest thing to a martyr for English science was Sir Francis Bacon, who died of a bad cold after stuffing an eviscerated goose with snow. Not even Galileo gave up his life to dispel the darkness of superstition. It took a poorly-educated schoolteacher in a remote and dusty town in South Africa to pay the ultimate price as a witness to natural causality. Professor Dawkins ought to be bursting with pride.

Or was he a martyr for his Christian faith? Of course he was, which is why the good Prof wouldn't dream of attending Sunday's festivities.

That's a mistake. Benedict Daswa's death is a dramatic demonstration that Christian faith and science do not conflict at all, but support each other. In fact, Christianity endorses the notion of an ordered, intelligible universe governed by its own rules. As John Paul II put it in a poetic epigram, "Faith and reason are like two wings on which the human spirit rises to the contemplation of truth."

The only incurable thing is the will to live!
MercatorNet, 4 March 2016

An Italian doctor who requires full-time care is still a high achiever

Monday, February 29, was Rare Disease Day, an international initiative to promote awareness of the thousands of crippling disorders. It's a good opportunity to highlight how courageously their victims deal with adversity.

It would hard to find a better example of this than the new chairman of the board of Italy's peak body for regulating pharmaceutical products, Agenzia italiana del Farmaco (AIFA), Mario Melazzini.

Melazzini was appointed by the Minister of Health in January, after his predecessor resigned over conflict of interest issues. He was an unusual choice. For about 20 years he practiced as a cancer specialist. But for the last 14 years he has suffered from Amyotrophic Lateral Sclerosis (ALS or Lou Gehrig's disease), the same ailment as the famous theoretical physicist Stephen Hawking.

He has to use a ventilator to breath properly; he needs a wheelchair for mobility; he is fed intravenously; and he needs constant care.

Despite all this, he has ticked off an impressive list of achievements. He is president of Aris, the Italian research foundation for ALS; he is a former councillor for health and research in the region of Lombardy, and he is the author of five books about disability, euthanasia and his own wrestling match with ALS.

His latest book was published late last year, *Lo sguardo e la speranza: La vita è bella, non solo nei film* (*The look and the hope: life is beautiful, and not just in the movies*). The title, a sly reference to the Oscar-winning Italian film *Life is Beautiful*, sums up his own philosophy of life.

He recently explained what he meant in an interview with Business International, an Italian magazine:

> When I started to look at my disease with fresh eyes, I understood it and made a fresh start on life. The moment I stopped thinking about what I could not do because of ALS, but what I could still do for myself, for my children and friends, my life changed ...
>
> "Life is a gift, an asset which must be nurtured from the moment of conception to natural end, even with illness. Life must not be manipulated according to an ideology. We need to realise that in any condition, when properly supported, everything can be seen as a great opportunity ... The only incurable thing is the will to live!

This optimism has been hard-won. In the months after he was diagnosed with ALS in 2002, he felt that his life was not worth living. He was becoming completely dependent on other people. He had lost weight and could eat and drink only with great difficulty. A PEG tube had been inserted into his stomach to feed him. There had been medical crises.

One day in 2003 he typed "assisted suicide" into a search engine and found Dignitas, a Swiss clinic which helps foreigners to die in Zurich. He rang them and made an appointment – but eventually decided not to go. He began to realise that life was too beautiful and precious.

His "conversion" influenced a heated debate over assisted

suicide in Italy in 2006. Another man with a degenerative disease, 61-year-old Piergiorgio Welby, was campaigning for the right to die. As a spokesman for victims of neurodegenerative disease and as a doctor, Melazzini campaigned for the right to life.

His participation in public life is a remarkable effort for a man who is so physically limited.

Melazzini's Catholic faith has sustained him throughout his illness, especially by reading the Old Testament book of Job, the just man stripped of everything he loved and owned. But his expectation of miracles is modest – not the miracle of a cure, but the miracle of acceptance:

> The miracle is not walking, drinking and many other things that I can no longer do. The miracle is serenity and an awareness of my limitations. I can't ask for anything more than what I had. I thought that I would be dead after a few years of illness, and instead, here I am, alive and active…
>
> The miracle happened: I opened my heart. I was locked into myself. Now I am open to myself and this allowed me to open up wide to others.

He says that he has been very influenced by Fr Luigi Giussani, the founder of an important Catholic group called Comunione e Liberazione. From him he learned that even with his immobility, he was still free. "With all my problems I was still happy." His Christian outlook gave him hope:

"Hope [he writes in *Lo Sguardo e la Speranza*] is a path that can lead to a better space. Pain and suffering, as such, are neither good nor desirable – but that doesn't mean that they are meaningless. And suffering can be contextualised and treated as a life experience."

He concludes the book with a remarkable idea: that sickness of the body can restore a sick soul to health:

> In our day-to-day lives, all of us will meet suffering sooner or later, and not just physical pain, sickness and frailty. We ought to be able to treasure it, turning it into something valuable in our path through life... And the disease can really become a form of health. It's healthy because it allows us to feel useful again for ourselves and for others, beginning with the family and including friends and colleagues. It's healthy because it helps us to realise that in life one should never take anything for granted, not even a glass of water sipped without choking.

It's an impressive story of a brave and wise man, though marred by his decision to split with Daniela, the wife who had cared for him and borne his three children. Last year he married Monica, a divorced woman with two children of his own whom he had met through the ALS association.

Divorce, of course, is forbidden by his Church, so the couple had to be married in a garden by a local official, not in a church. But in one of those baffling inconsistencies that bedevil our nature, Melazzini remains an enthusiastic Catholic.

Oh well. Even heroes are human.

Part 4
The miserabilists

The great human dignity heist

In the bittersweet song in "Fiddler on the Roof" Tevye sings "Be happy! Be healthy! Long life! / And if our good fortune never comes, Here's to whatever comes. / Drink l'chaim, to life!". Many of the leading figures in contemporary bioethics would refuse to sing "l'chaim, to life!" Not only are they not pro-life, they are not pro joie de vivre, which may be something even more serious. As one bioethicist puts it, citing a Yiddish jest, "Life is so terrible, it would have been better never to have been born. Who is so lucky? Not one in a hundred thousand!" A fundamental principle of bioethics based on human dignity is that life, with all of its limitations, is a good thing, a thing to be treasured. The miserabilist strain in bioethics denies this.

Who's the miserabilist of them all?
Spiked, 7 November 2007

There is stiff competition these days for the title of 'Biggest Misanthrope'. But with his 'pro-death' book on why it is better never to have been born, David Benatar is definitely in the lead.

What is it about utilitarians that makes them such miserabilists? The greatest happiness for the greatest number is the heart of their philosophy, but just try to find a happy utilitarian. The first of them, Jeremy Bentham, was such a sourpuss that he seemed pickled in vinegar. And in fact, he was, sort of. His embalmed body still sits in a cabinet in University College London, one of its principal tourist attractions. He had no wife and no children.

Herbert Spencer, a mutton-chopped Victorian who seems to be enjoying a quiet revival nowadays amongst sociobiologists, used utilitarianism to create a colossal metaphysical system. But the nearest he came to romance was a friendship with the rather horsey-looking George Eliot. In his early thirties he had a nervous breakdown and spent the rest of his long life as a hypochondriac semi-hermit wearing earplugs to avoid trivial conversation. And while Peter Singer, the most notorious of contemporary utilitarians, may be a karaoke champ in private life, his writings suggest otherwise.

However, these are bit players in the drama of miserabilism compared with South African academic David Benatar, author of *Better Never to Have Been: The Harm of Coming into Existence*. Although the book has not been widely reviewed in the popular press, it was published by Oxford University Press and has been presented as a serious contribution to the increasingly influential philosophy of utilitarianism.

Professor Benatar's thesis is that life is so horrid that we all would be better off had we never existed. And not just us, but all sentient life. He introduces his thesis with a Jewish witticism: 'Life is so terrible; it would have been better never to have been born. Who is so lucky? Not one in a hundred thousand!'

But Benatar is serious. 'The central idea of this book is that coming into existence is always a serious harm.' And, he continues, 'Coming into existence is always bad for those who come into existence. In other words, although we may not be able to say of the never-existent that never existing is good for them, we can say of the existent that existence is bad for them.'

How does he reach this conclusion, which, even by his own reckoning, seems absurd and repellent? As a utilitarian, he calculates the benefits of existence by balancing benefits against harms. What possible benefit could a non-existent person receive that would outweigh a pinprick of pain? Since most people find this hard to accept, Benatar spends a chapter demonstrating that 'human lives contain much more bad than is ordinarily recognised'.

Given his distaste for life, why has he hung around for so long? It's hard to say. Perhaps he agrees with American writer Dorothy Parker:

> Razors pain you, Rivers are damp,
> Acids stain you, And drugs cause cramp.
> Guns aren't lawful, Nooses give,
> Gas smells awful. You might as well live.

As you might expect, the extinction of the human race seems like an excellent idea to Prof B, although he acknowledges that it might be difficult for society to manage it in a humane fashion. However, if a couple of asteroids could be coaxed into colliding with our planet, it would be a positive outcome for all concerned.

The 19th-century German Arthur Schopenhauer is generally reckoned the most pessimistic of all philosophers, but in Benatar he has no mean rival. For the South African academic has more than a philosophy – he has a practical bioethical programme. Although, as a libertarian, he acknowledges that people have a right to have children, he feels that it is generally unethical, since it brings them into a world of harm. Supporters of abortion contend that women have a moral right to have abortions, but Prof B begs to differ: they have a moral obligation to have abortions, lest they add to the total amount of suffering in the world. Needless to say, this applies to animals, too. He describes his standpoint, somewhat defiantly, not as pro-choice, but as 'pro-death'.

Philosophers have often inspired poets. Epicurus had Lucretius; Thomas Aquinas had Dante; Shaftesbury had Pope; Kant had Coleridge; Mme Blavatsky had Yeats. But I can't think of a poet who could bear to warble on about Professor Benatar's vision. Perhaps the novelist HG Wells comes closest. In his classic *The Time Machine*, the Time Traveller goes so far into the future that all life is extinct:

> All the sounds of man, the bleating of sheep, the cries of birds, the hum of insects, the stir that makes the background of our lives – all that was over. As the darkness thickened, the eddying flakes grew more abundant, dancing before my eyes; and the cold of the air more intense. At last, one by one, swiftly, one after the other, the white peaks of the distant hills vanished into blackness. The breeze rose to a moaning wind. I saw the black central shadow of the eclipse sweeping towards me. In another

moment the pale stars alone were visible. All else was rayless obscurity. The sky was absolutely black.

Sounds like a great place to send Prof B for his Christmas holiday.

Benatar's bleak pessimism would be comic if it were not so widely shared amongst the woollier sort of environmentalists. *The World Without Us*, for instance, explores how long it would take for the human footprint to be washed away by the effluxion of time – about 500 years, it seems, although the good news is that plastic bags will hang around for a few million years. Meanwhile, a morbid fascination with a suicidally shrinking population seems to hold groups like the Optimum Population Trust in its thrall.

Tim Flannery, science's answer to Stephen King, insists that the population Down Under (where I live) should contract from 20 million to an optimum level of six million to keep us from wreaking havoc upon the environment. He was named 2007 Australian of the Year, so his message seems to have struck a chord amongst the extra-skinny soy latté set, at least. And judging from the hectoring of the United Nations Population Fund and its gaggle of birth control busybody NGOs, nearly everyone in Africa, Asia and South America urgently needs condoms to keep brown babies from entering the world and, later on, from entering Europe.

As one Amazon reviewer of *Better Never to Have Been* pointed out, 'you need a PhD to be this stupid'. Benatar's pessimism is the blind elaboration of the central utilitarian thesis: that good is a balance of pleasure and pain. But everyday life gives the lie to this. Utility is a soulless way to assess happiness and to know what is good. You don't have to be a martyr to realise that the pain of raising children is amply compensated by their love. Or that the pain of work is outweighed by the joy of achievement.

Or that a sunrise over Everest obliterates the pain of climbing there.

Are these watertight refutations? No, and, to be fair, Benatar deserves a few rounds of philosophical fisticuffs with a fellow academic. But common sense is enough for me. The great Samuel Johnson was once challenged to counter Berkeley's theory that matter was a figment of our imagination: 'I never shall forget', says his biographer Boswell, 'the alacrity with which Johnson answered, striking his foot with mighty force against a large stone, till he rebounded from it, "I refute it THUS".'

Nonetheless, *Better Never to Have Been* has its own modest utility. It unveils 'the greatest good of the greatest number' as the secret password of nihilism. And it is a lesson in intellectual history: after two centuries, the bitter streams gushing from Bentham and Spencer have finally trickled into the Dead Sea of the University of Cape Town philosophy department. Anyone toying with the seductive arguments of Peter Singer and his ilk should read it. There they will see what happens when the precepts of utilitarianism are taken to their logical conclusions.

A victor in wars which haven't happened

MercatorNet, 13 October 2007

> *The real problem with this year's Nobel Peace Prize is the canonisation of the precautionary principle.*

No award confers a greater guarantee of integrity and moral seriousness than the Nobel Peace Prize. Now Al Gore, former US Vice-President, former presidential candidate, Oscar winner and soothsayer of climate change, has ascended to the pantheon of Alfred Nobel's peacemakers. There he joins luminaries like Albert Schweitzer, the Dalai Lama, Mother Teresa, Martin Luther King and Andrei Sakharov.

The Norwegian Nobel Committee was certainly courting controversy when it garlanded Gore and the Intergovernmental Panel on Climate Change (IPCC). Its decision has been interpreted as a two-fingered salute to George Bush, an endorsement of dubious science or truckling to the greenies. But this is unfair: the Peace Prize has always been provocative.

Statesmen were controversial choices from the start. In 1906, the committee awarded it to Teddy Roosevelt for his role in bringing an end to the Russo-Japanese War of 1905. He is one of America's greatest presidents, but also a benevolent imperialist whose motto was "speak softly and carry a big stick". Since Norway had only become independent from Sweden in 1905, journalists interpreted the decision as a quiet plea for "a large, friendly neighbour — even if he is far away."

And interfering in domestic politics is nothing new either. In 1935, on the eve of World War II, it was awarded to Carl von

Ossietzky, a German journalist in a Nazi concentration camp for his opposition to German re-armament. It had never before been awarded to a person who opposed his own government's policies. A Norwegian newspaper at the time even protested that "a lasting peace between peoples and nations can only be achieved by respecting the existing laws". In hindsight, the committee made an admirable and courageous choice. (Ossietzky died in prison in 1938.)

The odd thing about this year's award is not its controversy, but that the laureates have done nothing for peace. The 2004 laureate, Kenyan Wangari Maathai, was also an environmentalist, but at least she was an activist for women's rights. When it comes to fighting for peace, Gore and the IPCC haven't done a blessed thing. They haven't even talked about doing a blessed thing. So the real laureate for 2007 is the "precautionary principle" -- sometime, somewhere, something awful might happen. This is clear from the text of the Prize press release:

> Extensive climate changes may alter and threaten the living conditions of much of mankind. They may induce large-scale migration and lead to greater competition for the earth's resources. Such changes will place particularly heavy burdens on the world's most vulnerable countries. There may be increased danger of violent conflicts and wars, within and between states.

Isn't there something a bit loopy about canonising the precautionary principle? Poor old Immanuel Velikovsky died too soon. He would have joined the pantheon for warning humanity of the danger of collisions with asteroids. You can just imagine the political upheaval which may occur if one of them flattens Oslo.

So many catastrophes are waiting to happen nowadays. Calamities are everywhere, each with its scenario of human rights violations, increased competition and wars. The terrifying consequences of the obesity epidemic, stranger danger, the depression epidemic, decreasing biodiversity, discrimination against homosexuals, religious fundamentalism and not flossing your teeth have yet to be explored by the Peace Prize Committee.

Granting Nobel Prizes for averting disasters which might happen is a sign that the committee is running out of ideas about peace. It was not always thus. In 1997, it awarded the prize to the International Campaign to Ban Landmines and its coordinator Jody Williams. Is it blind to the long list of genuine causes in the same vein? Trafficking of women? Treatment of refugees? Forced abortions? Religious oppression? Surely campaigners against these ghastly realities are persons who, as Nobel stipulated, "shall have done the most or the best work for fraternity between nations, for the abolition or reduction of standing armies and for the holding and promotion of peace congresses".

Perhaps the fundamental problem with the Nobel Peace Prize is the philosophy which inspires it. It assumes that lasting peace can be achieved through political activism and improved technology.

Nobel was a religious sceptic, a child of the Enlightenment who believed that technological progress was human progress. He even believed that dynamite, the invention which made his fortune, would end wars. In 1891, 23 years before the slaughter of World War I, he wrote to peace activist Bertha von Suttner that "Perhaps my factories will put an end to war sooner than your congresses: on the day that two army corps can mutually annihilate each other in a second, all civilised nations will surely recoil with horror and disband their troops."

The folly of this has been proved over and over again in the 20th Century. Handing an award to climate change whistleblowers simply perpetuates the error of thinking that there will be lasting peace without a clear conception of justice and a shared vision of truth.

Time to throw in the towel

MercatorNet, 8 September 2008

The ideas of a well-established bioethicist are so weird that it makes one despair of bioethics itself.

If you thought Peter Singer, now a professor at Princeton University, was Australia's gift to world bioethics, then I have news for you. One of his PhD students, now a professor at Oxford, Julian Savulescu, is leaving him in the dust.

While Singer is famed for supporting animal liberation, infanticide, euthanasia, and so on, Savulescu has broken new ground. A youthful 44, he has been at Oxford since 2002 as the head of something called the Uehiro Centre for Practical Ethics.

His postal address may be an ivory tower but he gets down and dirty with "practical ethics". He argues trenchantly for performance enhancing drugs in sport, genetic screening, early abortion, late-term abortion, sex-selective abortion, embryonic stem cell research, hybrid embryos, saviour siblings, therapeutic cloning, reproductive cloning, genetic engineering of children for higher IQs, eugenics, and organ markets.

For starters.

What is more, the sporty, good-looking, energetic Professor Savulescu has been fabulously successful in securing funding to promote his theories. He recently received a £800,000 (A$1.7 million) grant to investigate the ethics of tinkering with the brain. In short, to quote Oxford University, Julian Savulescu is internationally recognized as "a world-class bioethicist".

And back home in his native Melbourne, he is a minor media celebrity. A couple of years ago he even addressed the National Press Club. This gives great weight to his views on abortion. The state of Victoria is in the middle of a heated debate over the legalisation of abortion. The government supports it, but is studying how far to go. Should it merely decriminalise it? Should it legalise "a woman's choice" up to 24 weeks? Should it legalise abortion at any stage in a pregnancy? There is no doubt about where Savulescu stands: "Abortion is a legitimate way for people to control the number of children they have," he said the other day.

Which provokes me to suggest something even more radical than his outlandish theories. After several years of reviewing the theories of Savulescu and his colleagues, I'm fed up. It's time to abolish bioethics and bioethicists. What we need is plain vanilla ethics.

That sexy little prefix "bio" has become a Kevlar vest for so-called experts who couldn't score a job in the philosophy department of Monty Python's University of Woolloomooloo. Because there is no agreement about what bioethics is, about what areas it should cover, or about its fundamental principles, just about anyone can dub themselves a bioethicist. And just about anyone does.

The word "bioethics" was only coined in the 60s or 70s. Forty years on, we have progressive bioethics, conservative bioethics, global bioethics, feminist bioethics, Islamic bioethics, Catholic bioethics, utilitarian bioethics, deontological bioethics, dignitarian bioethics (my favourite), and so on. Bioethics, as most of the real experts quietly agree, is a field in crisis. Jonathan Moreno, one of America's leading bioethicists, has spoken of "a crisis of identity" and questioned "the survival of bioethics as we have known it".

The point is, what makes the theories of bioethicists like Julian Savulescu's credible? Are they consistent with common sense, with human nature, with sound public policy? Why should we believe them rather than television evangelists or New Age gurus? The problem is broader than Savulescu or Singer. A growing number of influential bioethicists are defending bizarre theories in leading journals and getting funding to bring them into mainstream debate.

It might interest Victorian parliamentarians, for instance, to know that Savulescu has a shadow life as a New Age guru who gushes about the loopy theory of transhumanism. "People have predicted there'll be a huge spike in computing power and artificial intelligence," he told a newspaper not long ago. "At some point this century people could upload into machines." You can read all about it in his upcoming book, "Enhancement of Human Beings".

My hunch is that Savulescu's prestige is based on the cachet of his Oxford appointment and his prodigious capacity for work. Not on his ideas. Far from being sophisticated and profound, all of Savulescu's arguments run on the same rails. Why shouldn't we do transgressive action X? he demands. X hurts no one. X is an expression of autonomy. X is my right. Do you object that X is against human nature? No such thing, buddy. Therefore, X is ethical. Let us, then, be courageously transgressive.

It's all very logical. And it steamrollers common sense.

I confess that I have not read all of the articles in Professor Savulescu's 21-page curriculum vitae, but I suspect that 90 per cent of them follow this playbook.

As confirmation of this, I sampled his views on apotemnophilia, a psychiatric condition whose sufferers are obsessed with a desire to amputate perfectly healthy limbs. True bioethicists love this sort of weirdness. What does Savulescu have to say? It comes straight from his playbook: "Thus not only might amputation be permissible; in some situations, it might be desirable. While it is a tragedy for nearly all of us to lose a limb, there might be good reasons for certain rare individuals to choose this fate. We must be open to such radical possibilities."

Now, if Professor Savulescu were a mere philosopher, rather than an Oxford Bioethicist, he would be laughed offstage. To paraphrase George Orwell, some ideas are so stupid that only a bioethicist could promote them. Professor Savulescu certainly has a high IQ, but more than logic is needed to pontificate about apotemnophilia, or abortion, for that matter. You need common sense, a breadth of experience and a deep and sympathetic appreciation of human nature. In short, you need to be a plain vanilla ethicist.

The science of morality

Australasian Science, November 2010

A leading researcher into the biological basis of morality has been found guilty of academic misconduct.

Morality is a tricky business. If you are an expert, people tend to hold you to a higher standard of probity. That's why sex abuse scandals and the double lives of televangelists have done such damage to the cause of religious morality. Perhaps, too, this is why academic misconduct by one of the leading exponents of the "new science of morality" has rattled scientists and bioethicists.

In August, Harvard University announced that a popular lecturer, 51-year-old Professor Marc D. Hauser, was guilty of eight instances of unspecified scientific misconduct, three involving published papers and five unpublished material. "There were problems involving data acquisition, data analysis, data retention, and the reporting of research methodologies and results," a university official admitted. Harvard has resisted pressure to reveal the dreary details, but the word on the academic grapevine is that Hauser may have performed experiments without a control group, making them utterly useless.

"If it's the case the data have in fact been fabricated, which is what I as the editor infer, that is as serious as it gets," said the editor of *Cognition,* Gerry Altmann, who has withdrawn a 2002 paper of which Hauser was the lead author.

Hauser's future is uncertain. The case is being investigated by the Federal government as it may involve misuse of research funds. He has taken a year's leave of absence and told the *New*

York Times that "I acknowledge that I made some significant mistakes," and that he was "deeply sorry for the problems this case had caused to my students, my colleagues and my university".

Academic misconduct seldom makes headlines, but Hauser's case is different. His interests extended far beyond whether tamarind monkeys can recognise themselves in a mirror. He was a leading figure in the "new science of morality", a movement that argues persuasively that right and wrong are based on biologically determined gut feelings, not reason. It is a revolutionary effort to wrest right and wrong from the pulpit and plonk it on the lab bench.

Earlier this year a high-profile conference brought together some of the movement's leading lights. Along with Hauser there was Jonathan Haidt, whose theory is that modern morality is based on primal feelings of disgust, and another Harvard professor, Joshua D. Greene, who argues that it is an anachronistic hangover from the Palaeolithic era.

Hauser has been deeply influenced by the controversial linguist Noam Chomsky, and believes that morality is like language. Just as there is a universal grammar, with particular applications, there is a universal capacity for moral thinking, but each culture has its own moral toolkit. That is why we all profess to be moral but we find each other's moral codes incomprehensible.

This approach has unsettling consequences for the man in the street. If my morality and the morality of Pathan tribesmen in Afghanistan are as different as English and Pushtu, how can I say that female genital mutilation is wrong? Nor is banning abortion any more "reasonable" than Chinese is more "reasonable" than Spanish.

Nor does morality have any link to transcendent values. As

Hauser wrote in his 2006 book, *Moral Minds*, the "marriage between morality and religion is not only forced but unnecessary, crying out for a divorce".

But how can Hauser's troubles discredit the new science of morality? To err is human, and disgraced preachers haven't discredited the doctrines of Christianity. Up to a point, this is obviously true.

But Hauser and his colleagues are not just the preachers but the founders of a new approach to morality. And it is a stand that has many followers among bioethicists. If biology explains morality, then objections to stem cell research, abortion and euthanasia, for instance, are based on nothing more substantial than the "yuck factor". In 2010 it's time to rip up the Palaeolithic rule book and write our own.

Unhappily, Hauser's misstep suggests that the founders might not even respect their own rule books. "I believe that science, and scientists, have an important role to play in shaping the moral agenda. We have an obligation to use facts and reason to guide what we ought to do," Hauser contended forcefully in a recent essay on *The Edge*.

Well, facts and reason didn't stop him from stooping to academic misconduct. No big deal, perhaps, in comparison to murder or torture but it does make one hesitate to hand over the future of morality to Harvard professors. Who knows what barriers they might breach next?

Hauser's next book is said to be titled *Evilicious: Explaining Our Evolved Taste for Being Bad*. It will make interesting reading.

Even more weirdness
MercatorNet, 20 March 2012

Are all bioethicists crazy? Or only the utilitarians?

Newspapers have their "silly season" of shock-horror absurdities in the slow news summer months. How about bioethics journals? When two very loopy articles in peer-reviewed journals surface in as many weeks, their silly season is clearly February and March.

First two Italian/Australians asserted in the *Journal of Medical Ethics* that infanticide was morally permissible. That created a firestorm of commentary which badly tarnished the prestige of bioethics as a serious discipline.

Now an American, a Swede and a Briton are about to publish an even weirder article in a journal called *Environment, Ethics and Policy*. Their proposal is to combat climate change with human engineering. People who are smaller and shorter and eat less meat will help reduce both their own carbon footprint and bovine flatulence (which is a significant contributor to greenhouse gases).

The details of their essay are so extraordinary that some caveats are needed to ensure that the authors get a fair hearing. First of all, although engineering children is clearly eugenics, the authors insist that it is the nice kind of eugenics, the privatised voluntary kind, not the government-enforced mandatory kind.

Second, these are thought experiments, not practical proposals. And third, the eccentricity of the solutions is justified by the urgency of the problem. International agreements on carbon emissions are not working and the feasibility of geo-engineering the planet by changing the chemistry of the oceans or sucking carbon dioxide out of the atmosphere with giant sponges seems remote.

So imaginative solutions are needed – which the three bioethicists, who come from New York University and from Oxford, supply. In spades.

Their most eye-popping brainwave is turning us into hobbits. "For instance," one author, S. Matthew Liao, of New York University, told *The Atlantic*, "if you reduce the average U.S. height by just 15cm, you could reduce body mass by 21% for men and 25% for women, with a corresponding reduction in metabolic rates by some 15% to 18%, because less tissue means lower energy and nutrient needs."

Another intriguing proposal is inducing positive attitudes towards the environment with drugs, although Liao sees it as a way of boosting willpower rather than inducing beliefs.

> If you crave steak, and that craving prevents you from making a decision you otherwise want to make, in some sense your inability to control yourself is a limit on the will, or a limit on your liberty. A meat patch would allow you to truly decide whether you want to have that steak or not, and that could be quite liberty enhancing.

Then there is population control. Liao dismisses the one-child policy advocated by some environmental groups as coercive. He favours a child-per-family quota based on volume and weight rather than number. Parents could have three small-sized children or two medium-sized children or one really large basketball player.

Preposterous?

Don't be too quick to judge. Another author, Rebecca Roache, of Oxford told the Guardian that most great ideas often seem preposterous at first.

> Human engineering may seem bizarre and unrealistic, but this does not mean it could not turn out to be feasible and promising: telephones, 'test tube babies', and personal computers are all important aspects of modern life that were once regarded as bizarre and unrealistic.

The article has even been criticised by other bioethicists, the Swedish author, Anders Sandberg, admitted to *The Guardian*. But he is unperturbed by labels like "eco-Nazis" and "eugenicists". "We are fairly typical liberal academics thinking about the world," Sandburg says.

Well, if Liao, Roache and Sandberg are typical, there is something wrong with liberal academics. They have blithely overlooked so many social, political and moral objections and have such a feeble grasp on what makes us human that they bring all of bioethics into disrepute – just as the authors of the infanticide paper did.

What is the source of these common-sense defying conjectures? After all, writing science fiction is not part of an ordinary bioethicist's job description. Most of them are busy chipping away at the coal face, clarifying the conundrums that crop up every day of a doctor's life. It's simply not true that bioethics is one of "the world's most unnecessary occupations", along with aroma therapists, golf pros, journalism professors and American vice-presidents, as Andrew Ferguson sneered recently in *The Weekly Standard*.

As bioethics blogger Wesley J. Smith points out, we owe a lot to bioethicists who think deeply about the problems arising from technological mastery over the human body. Thinkers like Leon Kass or Gilbert Meilander or Margaret Somerville have helped to clarify the issues.

Respectable bioethicists can be controversial, but only a few have slipped their moorings from common sense and floated off to la-la land. These are the academics who are regularly pilloried in the media. Where do they come from?

My hunch is that most media wildfires are lit by utilitarians. If you examine the academic credentials of the five academics involved in these recent papers, all of them had links with Oxford and/or Monash University in Melbourne, both redoubts of utilitarianism. The notorious Peter Singer worked for many years at Monash, and his student, Julian Savulescu, now heads up the Uehiro Centre for Practical Ethics at Oxford.

You might think that utilitarianism, whose foundational principle is the greatest good for the greatest number, is a left-brain theory for bean-counters. The first utilitarian, the 19th century philosopher Jeremy Bentham, taught that the most ethical solution could be reached with his "felicific calculus" – balancing pleasures and pains without need for any transcendent realities.

But there is a right-brain side to this dry-as-dust philosophy. Highly logical people are often drawn to weird forms of spirituality. Jeremy Bentham, for instance, is a beacon of incandescent weirdness for succeeding generations. He specified in his will that his body was to be preserved, dressed in his best clothes, and displayed in a glass cabinet to inspire "pilgrims [and] votaries of the greatest-happiness principle". For years before his death – so it is said -- he jangled in his pockets the glass eyes which were to adorn his mummified skull. It was an odd way to become immortal.

One of the most significant theorists of utilitarianism, the 19th century philosopher Henry Sidgwick, also founded a Society for Psychical Research, which conducted sympathetic investigations into spiritualism – séances, communications with the dead and so on.

The miserabilists

Utilitarians don't believe in human nature, but only in a sliding scale of consciousness. Persons are beings (animal or human) who are capable of anticipating the future and of having wants and desires for the future. There is nothing stable and unchanging about human nature. So utilitarians are free to redefine what human beings are and what they can be. The less adventurous ones, like Peter Singer, are content to include some animals and to exclude infants and comatose adults. The more ambitious ones, like Julian Savulescu, an Oxford bioethicist, dream of enhancing our present condition with drugs and genetic engineering.

Moving to another level, there are transhumanists who have visions of Humanity 2.0. These humans of the future will be stronger and faster, vastly more intelligent and even more altruistic and peaceful. Some fantasise about achieving immortality by uploading their minds onto computers. This is a logical extension of the utilitarian mindset. If the boundaries of the future are not set by human nature, humanity is just a work in progress, a plaything for imaginative bioethicists.

Strictly speaking, transhumanists are not utilitarians, but utilitarian axioms underpin transhumanism. As Savulescu told an ethics journal a couple of years ago, the two approaches make a nice fit:

> Transhumanism has a kind of group-think or quasi-religious quality that does not suit well my nature. I prefer to stand outside it and make my own arguments. But their hearts (and minds) are in the right place. We agree on most things.

Despite the prestige that Singer and Savulescu and other utilitarians have, at least in the media, loopiness is hard-wired into their philosophy. A utilitarian bioethicist is always going to be a loose cannon, rolling wildly around the deck in ethical storms, splintering and smashing the fragile public image of his or her profession. If other bioethicists want to repair their dented prestige, shunning utilitarian colleagues would be a good place to start.

Part 5
Torture and other utilitarian games

Utilitarianism — the greatest good for the greatest number — is the default starting point for much discourse about bioethics. If destroying embryos leads to miracle cures for millions, why not? If euthanasia brings relief in a life which is more pain than pleasure, why not? If distributing condoms stops AIDS, why not?

The attractive thing about the utilitarianism of Peter Singer and a host of other bioethicists is its façade of steely logic. With geometric rigour, they argue from easily-grasped first principles to clearly defined conclusions. But it may surprise some people to learn that utilitarianism can also justify torture. If there is a ticking bomb hidden somewhere in a city, surely police are allowed to torture one bomb-maker if thousands of innocent lives can be saved.

But hang on! Isn't there something wrong with a philosophy which allows human rights to be violated in such an egregious way? This is a question which needs to be put to utilitarian sophists who offer easy solutions to complex and subtle human dilemmas.

The torture-abortion nexus

MercatorNet, 2 February 2015

Why do philosophers who defend abortion also defend torture?

Is there a necessary link between people who approve of abortion and people who approve of torture?

I can hear screams of denial. Abortion is a woman's right and has nothing to do with putting needles under fingernails. Abortion is an agonising choice by thoughtful women and has nothing to do with the agonies of waterboarding. And so on.

But how, then, are we to account for the fact that some of the world's most eminent moral philosophers who published intricate arguments for abortion in the 1990s are publishing intricate arguments for torture 20 years later?

Exhibit A is Professor Jeff McMahan, who strongly defended the use of torture in the *New York Times* last week. If you can kill to protect innocent people, you can torture to protect them, he argued.

McMahan is an American who was recently appointed to a prestigious chair at Oxford University in the UK. His interests centre on the ethics of killing – issues like brain death, euthanasia, just wars, and abortion. In his 2002 book, *The Ethics of Killing: Problems at the Margins of Life*, presents a long defence of the morality of abortion and even infanticide. This is grounded on his belief that we are embodied minds and that what happens to the body is only significant in so far as it affects our personal identity. Hence he contends that an abortion before 20 weeks is not harming anyone because (so he says) the foetus has no awareness until then.

Balancing this bleak perspective on human life, curiously, are his tender-hearted views on animal life. He is a vegetarian and believes that humans should not eat meat because killing animals deprives them of valuable future life experiences which outweigh the pleasures of eating meat.

It is not merely humans who should give up their carnivorous habits, but other animals. In an op-ed in the *New York Times* in 2010 he said that carnivore species should be made extinct because of the pain that they inflict upon herbivores. "It would be instrumentally good if predatory animal species were to become extinct and be replaced by new herbivorous species, provided that this could occur without ecological upheaval involving more harm than would be prevented by the end of predation."

But lovers of the ox and the lamb must have been disconcerted to read, again in the *New York Times*, that Professor McMahon supports torture. Within limits, of course. Mafia toe-cutting is out, along with the amusements of serial killers and the waterboarding used by the CIA in the bad old Bush days. But when push comes to shove, the gloves are off. "Torture can be morally justifiable, and even obligatory, when it is wholly defensive – for example, when torturing a wrongdoer would prevent him from seriously harming innocent people."

The reasoning for approving of torture has much in common with his argument for abortion and vegetarianism: "It can be morally justifiable to kill a person to prevent him from detonating a bomb that will kill innocent people, or to prevent him from killing an innocent hostage. Since being killed is generally worse than being tortured, it should therefore be justifiable to torture a person to prevent him from killing innocent people." In all these instances, McMahon balances pain against positive life experience.

Exhibit B is Frances Kamm, a stellar professor at Harvard University, in the US. One of the books that made her reputation as an ingenious moral philosopher was *Creation and Abortion*, published in 1992. Not one to resile from difficult conclusions, she concedes that even if the foetus is a person, abortion can be permissible. One of her arguments compares the benefits and cost to the foetus and its creator, the mother. If the foetus benefits by gaining life, it ought to bear some of the risk of being harmed or aborted. She writes, given our "strong reasons to reproduce, demanding complete security for the foetus seems unreasonable." It's not quite fair to reduce her chapters to a sentence-long grab, but perhaps this sums it up: "if the foetus will die without the woman's aid, and if she has no duty to aid it at a high cost to herself, then she may kill it if that is necessary to avoid the cost of aiding it."

So is it any surprise that Kamm pulled out the same philosophical scales in her recent book *Ethics for Enemies: Terror, Torture, and War*. In it she contends that torture may well be ethical. She writes, "it is sometimes permissible to torture someone, at least for a short time without permanent damage, if we would otherwise permissibly kill him". Another philosopher sums up her argument as follows:

> Her basic strategy is to say that in these situations it is permissible to *kill* people so as to prevent harm coming to other people, and then say that, because it is permissible to kill people so as to prevent harm coming to other people, it is permissible to torture people so as to prevent harm coming to other people – after all, they are better off tortured than killed!

This is clearly the same voice and the same mind which argued that unborn children can be killed. If babies can be killed for "threatening" the life, or even the mere interests, of the mother, why shouldn't suspected terrorists be tortured? (To be fair to

Kamm, she also argues that terrorism can sometimes be moral.)

So is there a link between abortion and torture? Most supporters of abortion will not march in demonstrations demanding torture for terrorists. Therefore it is not true to say that supporting abortion will lead the average person to support torture. But most supporters of abortion have never thought deeply about the arguments which underpin it, either. Those who have, like Jeff McMahan and Frances Kamm, recognise that supporting one necessarily leads to supporting the other.

Ivory tower arguments for torture in philosophy journals have real world consequences. McMahan relates that an American philosopher, Henry Slue, admitted that torture was not absolutely wrong in an influential article in 1978. Two CIA agents later thanked him. They were relieved to find that their day jobs were ethically justifiable.

Being "nice" worked in World War II. Why not now?

MercatorNet, 12 December 2014

Two legendary interrogators have lessons for the War on Terror

This week's Senate committee report on the involvement of the CIA in torture and mistreatment of detainees has exposed a bitter debate between human-rights-first interrogators and battle-hardened interrogators.

Former US Air Force Col. Steven Kleinman represents the human-right-first group. "As a career interrogator, I know that the lawful, humane methods for acquiring intelligence are also the most effective," he says. "Today's report only reinforces this fact and makes it publicly available to the American people. There is no need to debate this any longer. Now it's time to chart a new course for the future, one that will not only respect human rights, but will also keep America safe."

Now working as Director of Strategic Research at The Soufan Group, Kleinman backs his claims up with psychological research published in academic journals.

On the battle-hardened, whatever-it-takes side is Jason Beale, the pseudonym for an interrogator with years of experience in Iraq and Afghanistan. His bitter complaints about the Senate committee's investigation were published in The Weekly Standard in mid-November. Without naming him his words about Kleinman and his ilk were volcanic with rage.

> They are opportunists who, almost uniformly, spent a relatively

small portion of their professional lives engaged in standard interrogation be it criminal or intelligence-related and they bundled their manufactured credibility and their personal opinion into a nice little self-righteous quote package, for sale to the highest bidder.

Which side represents the old-school interrogator? Surprisingly, it could be Colonel Kleinman. In a sense, his tactics were proved effective during World War II, when the stakes were even higher than they are now in the War on Terror.

The High-Value Detainee Interrogation Group, an intelligence-gathering unit set up in 2010 by President Obama, recently released a publication outlining its philosophy. It's clear that two of the best interrogators in World War II have had a great influence on their approach.

One was a German, Hanns Joachim Scharff, a Luftwaffe interrogator who was so successful that some of the airmen whom he interrogated were tried for treason after the War because American authorities thought that they had willingly told the enemy everything.

The other was an American, Sherwood F. Moran, who interrogated Japanese prisoners at Guadalcanal. Moran's career is particularly interesting because he operated under conditions which were close to the "ticking bomb" scenario. Often he was speaking with prisoners who were still bleeding from wounds while under sniper fire and air bombardment. In 1944 he wrote some notes for interrogators which have become a classic in the intelligence community.

One of the secrets of his approach was that he treated the prisoner with the respect and dignity due to another human being.

> I often tell a prisoner right at the start what my attitude is! I

consider a prisoner (i.e. a man who has been captured and disarmed and in a perfectly *safe* place) as out of the war, out of the picture, and thus, in a way, not an enemy ... Notice that ... I used the word "safe." That is the point: get the prisoner to a safe place, where even he knows ... that it is all over. Then forget, as it were, the "enemy" stuff, and the "prisoner" stuff. I tell them to forget it, telling them I am talking as a human being to a human being.

The Japanese had a reputation for fanaticism and stubbornness. Yet by taking an interest in them as persons and treating them with concern, Moran managed to get them to share what they knew:

On [one] occasion a soldier was brought in. A considerable chunk of his shinbone had been shot away. In such bad shape was he that we broke off in the middle of the interview to have his leg redressed. We were all interested in the redressing, in his leg, it was almost a social affair! And the point to note is that we really *were* interested, and not pretending to be interested in order to get information out of him. This was the prisoner who called out to me when I was leaving after that first interview, "Won't you please come and talk to me *every day*." (And yet people are continually asking us, "Are the Japanese prisoners really willing to talk?")

But neither was Moran soft. He needed intelligence urgently during the Guadalcanal campaign. "Don't let your warm human interest, your genuine interest in the prisoner, cause you to be sidetracked by him! You should be hard-boiled but not half-baked. Deep human sympathy can go with a business-like, systematic and ruthlessly persistent approach."

Moran's background made him ideally suited for his job. He had been a Protestant missionary in Japan for more than 20 years and spoke the language perfectly. In 1948 he returned in Japan for another seven years of missionary work.

He brought his deep Christian virtues to the battlefield: mutual respect, cheerfulness, and hard work. His social work in Japan and his interrogation in Guadalcanal sprang from the same values; there was no disconnect. "He was probably the only Marine of his era who never took a drink, never smoked a cigarette, and never cursed. For their discipline and comradeship, he loved them like brothers," his family recalled in a memoir.

Nowadays the enemy is different; the style of warfare is different. What remains the same is the common humanity of the prisoner and the interrogator. What the experience of Sherwood F. Moran and others shows is that treating a captive as a fellow human being is not a soft option.

Does this work with all interrogators? What Moran thought may be surprising. For him, it was not a matter of exerting superior force, but of having "character", of being a man whom the prisoner will respect.

> Of course all this dignity emphasis is based on the fear that the prisoner will take advantage of you and your friendship; the same idea as that a foreman must swear at his construction gang in order to get work out of them. Of course there always is the danger that some types will take advantage of your friendliness. This is true in any phase of life, whether you are a teacher, a judge, an athletic trainer, a parent. But there is some risk in any method. But this is where the interpreter's character comes in, that I have so emphasized earlier in this article. You can't fool with a man of real character without eventually getting your fingers burned.

Was this the problem with the CIA interrogators? Did they lack that indefinable thing called character?

The guru of philanthropy

MercatorNet, 4 September 2009

Peter Singer's latest cause is lifting billions out of poverty.

If the wealthiest 10 percent of American families set aside at least 5 percent of their after-tax income, US$471 billion would be available each year to house, heal and feed the world's poorest 1.4 billion people. This is vastly greater than the US$189 billion a year needed to meet the Millennium Development goals -- the UN's targets for halving world poverty by 2015.

Hence, if people who suffer such dire poverty can be helped at the cost of so little sacrifice, it is morally depraved not to do so.

Such is the contention of Peter Singer, the world's most controversial philosopher, in his latest book, *The Life You Can Save: Acting Now To End World Poverty*. Singer is better known for supporting euthanasia and animal rights than for moonlighting as Mother Teresa. But his fans should not panic -- he uses the same principles to argue for both philanthropy and infanticide. I suspect that very few charitable foundations will be inviting him to join their boards of directors.

To his credit, for many years Singer has been a passionate advocate of a frugal lifestyle and philanthropy and a stern critic of the consumer society. He gives away 25 percent of his own income. As far back as 1972, he wrote an influential article, "Famine, Affluence, and Morality", which asked how it could be ethical to ignore the suffering of starving and diseased people. Singer seeks to shame Americans and citizens of other wealthy nations into digging deep. He cites heart-rending statistics to show that more people have died of preventable causes over the past 20 years than in all the wars and all the government repression of the bloody 20th century. It is deeply immoral, he says, to ignore this suffering.

His book concludes with a stirring quote from a man whose life has been a touchstone for Singer, animal liberationist Henry Spira:

> I guess basically one wants to feel that one's life has amounted to more than just consuming products and generating garbage. I think that one likes to look back and say that one's done the best one can to make this a better place for others. You can look at it from this point of view: what greater motivation can there be than doing whatever one possibly can to reduce pain and suffering?

Although *The life you can save* is rather skimpy on philosophy, it is an important book. It softens Singer's image as a brutal foe of human dignity and waves a magic wand over utilitarianism, transforming it into a philosophy of compassion, altruism and self-sacrifice. He even showcases utilitarian saints, people who have sacrificed large chunks of their income to help the poor. Is it a coincidence that the motto of the Bill & Melinda Gates Foundation, "All lives have equal value" is a fundamental axiom of Singer's philosophy?

One of Singer's heroes is Zell Kravinsky, an American who has two PhDs, has lectured on the poet Milton and has made a large fortune in Philadelphia real estate. Instead of wallowing in the sty of filthy lucre, he has given most of it away. He has but one suit, which he bought for $20 at a thrift shop. He even donated one of his kidneys to a stranger, ignoring his wife's objection that one of his children might need it someday. But, Kravinksky responded, "The sacrosanct commitment to the family is the rationalisation for all manner of greed and selfishness."

I suspect that Singer's sotto voce message is that Christianity (and other world religions) have failed to motivate people to live the Golden Rule, notwithstanding all their guff about human dignity. Utilitarianism is no less noble, and there's no guff.

However, when examined more closely, Singer's reasoning raises more questions than it answers.

First of all, it is not at all clear why a utilitarian should care about anyone else's welfare. With Singer it is axiomatic that we should relieve the suffering of other creatures. But why? What unites us? Why should I rescue a child drowning in six inches of water in a wading pool? And why should I be interested in the suffering of distant Africans? In a desperate attempt to show that we have a responsibility for helping Africans, Singer argues that each one of us has generated a proportion of greenhouse gases which bring drought and starvation. But even if this is true, it is not very motivating. Not for me, anyway.

Second, there is something chilling, even inhuman, about Singer's insistence that personal relationships are irrelevant. Another of his saints is a Harvard-educated doctor who works in Haiti, Paul Farmer. Farmer wrestles with the awful feeling that he is continually tempted to love his own child more than his patients. He calls it a "failure of empathy". If utilitarianism cannot account for a father's love for his own child, it's not much of a philosophy.

Third, whom are we obliged to help? After a while, it dawned on me that Singer is not interested in relieving the suffering of persons as individuals, but as members of crowds, as statistics. What motivates him is not charity, but irritation that resources are being deployed inefficiently. Besides, given what we know about Singer's interest in animal liberation, don't "all lives" include great apes, dogs, dolphins and pigs? They probably do, although it is hardly tactful to mention non-anthropoi in a tract about philanthropy.

In Singer's system, even "the joy of giving" is a dreary business. It may indeed give you joy, but his joy is just an evolved neurological response which lights up the brain's reward centres in MRI scans. As for the hungry Africans, once their immediate suffering has been relieved, I suspect that Singer will lose all interest. He has nothing more to offer. The things that bring meaning to most people's lives -- happiness, art, family ties -- are almost meaningless for him.

There is a curious inconsistency which runs through Singer's life and work. It is well known that he broke his own rules by caring generously for his mother after she was stricken with Alzheimer's disease. In some strange way, he seems to be constructing a philosophical foundation for Christian virtues like charity and self-sacrifice without admitting that human beings possess an inherent and inalienable dignity. But his clunky utilitarian calculus just doesn't work. I wonder just how successful he will be at inspiring people to abandon their iPods and yachts to save the poor.

A few weeks ago I was lucky enough to attend a packed lecture at Melbourne University by Singer to promote *The Life You Can Save*. His audience was goggle-eyed and the questions were more marshmallows than softballs. So I asked him one. What if you had to choose between feeding a dozen stranded dolphins and feeding a dozen brain-damaged infants with a low life expectancy? He looked quite irritated and didn't give a clear answer. So much for the philanthropy of our ascetical utilitarian guru.

Calculating charity

MercatorNet, 2 June 2015

Peter Singer's new book on philanthropy reveals a dark side to utilitarianism

Australian philosopher Peter Singer has been described as "a man of principles and towering intellect". Both qualities are at centre stage in his latest book, *The Most Good You Can Do: How Effective Altruism Is Changing Ideas About Living Ethically*.

Although he is better known as the leading theorist of animal liberation and for his controversial ideas about bioethics, philanthropy is one of Singer's passions. As early as 1972 he had already formulated most of the arguments which he showcases in this book and in a 2010 book, *The Life You Can Save: How to Do Your Part to End World Poverty*.

Doing the most good you can do with limited resources is an ethical challenge which utilitarianism is almost designed to handle. Input your resources, a community's needs and your personal preferences, press a button and the "felicific calculus" cranks out an ethical response. An interactive game on the book's website even displays a "charity impact calculator" which estimates how much your donation will buy when you give to a particular foundation.

Singer's idea is that we are ethically bound to be effectively altruistic. It is immoral to allow waste, to splurge on ourselves, or to support projects like museums which do nothing to lessen the world's misery.

This is great PR for utilitarianism, which has suffered from the perception that its adherents are crabby gentlemen with green eye-shades who are always doing cost-benefit analyses. *The Most Good That You Can Do* shows that utilitarians are not baked in the mould of Mr Gradgrind, Dickens' parody of a utilitarian in *Hard Times*. Like Christians, and even more than Christians, they take the wretched of the earth seriously. As a utilitarian, you can be altruistic without airy-fairy ideals. Even more, you can live with all the austerity of a Franciscan without believing in God, but with the satisfaction of witnessing that your generosity has bettered the lives of others.

His approach has stellar supporters. "An optimistic and compelling look at the positive impact that giving can have on the world," say Bill and Melinda Gates. "Singer's argument is powerful, provocative and, I think, basically right," says *New York Times* columnist Nicholas Kristoff.

But does this prove that utilitarianism is a sound moral guide through life's trackless wilderness? There is more to ethics than altruism. Does Singer handle other moral dilemmas convincingly?

Perhaps not.

There is a very, very peculiar passage in the book which Bill and Melinda appear not to have read. If they had, they would have thought twice about adopting Singer as the intellectual patron of their philanthropic foundation. If you had unearthed a letter of Martin Luther King Jr expressing his admiration for *Mein Kampf*, or an interview with Mother Teresa criticizing the poor for being dirty and stupid, you could not be more surprised.

What is an ethical career, Singer asks. This is a more difficult question than it seems at first blush. Working for Oxfam gets a tick. But how about for Goldman Sachs (or Microsoft)? That also

Torture and other utilitarian games

gets a tick. Why? Because you can distribute your high (or even obscenely high) salary according to the principles of effective altruism.

So far so good.

But when Singer asks whether someone can work for Goldman Sachs even if it supports an abomination like, say, tobacco companies, he comes up with an astonishing conclusion:

> For someone who judges actions by their consequences, to be complicit in wrongful harm requires that one make a difference to the likelihood of the harm occurring. As we saw earlier, if you do not take the position offered by the investment bank, someone else will, and from the bank's perspective that person will probably be nearly as good as you would have been. .... you may have a better chance of altering the bank's actions-or, through the bank, the actions of the corporation for which it is raising money-if you are on the inside than if you are protesting from outside.

This sounds very much like selling out to the system. "If I didn't do it, someone else would have," was an excuse often heard from Nazis after the War. And, astonishingly for a man with three grandparents who perished in the Holocaust, Singer pursues the logic of his position until he ends up defending the guards at Auschwitz.

> The consequentialist notion of complicity does have implications that many people will reject. It implies, for instance, that the guards at Auschwitz were not acting wrongly if their refusal to serve in that role would have led only to their replacement by someone else, perhaps someone who would have been even more brutal toward those who were about to be murdered there.
>
> Given that serving as a concentration camp guard was often an alternative to being sent to the Russian front, this hypothetical was probably sometimes true.

The great human dignity heist

> Strictly utilitarian effective altruists ... would have to accept the implication that, on a plausible reading of the relevant facts, at least some of the guards at Auschwitz were not acting wrongly.

Hang on. This violates all the moral intuitions of the average man. How many aged prison guards have been dragged before German courts in recent years and found guilty of complicity in Nazi atrocities, even if they did almost nothing?

"No man is an island" and somehow we are all complicit – perhaps to a very small degree – in the injustices which are part of our life stories. Otherwise, why should the US Senate have apologised for 200 years of slavery? Why should Australian Prime Minister Kevin Rudd have apologised for his nation's treatment of Aborigines? Why should John Paul II have apologised for the Crusades?

In fact, at this very moment an Auschwitz guard is on trial in Germany for complicity in the deaths of 300,000 Jews. He is a perfect fit for Singer's criteria for not acting wrongly.

Oskar Gröning, now 93, was the "bookkeeper of Auschwitz" from 1942 to 1944. He collected and counted the cash of people who had been exterminated. That's all. Somebody else would have done the job if he refused. Yet this excuse gave him little consolation. For the rest of his life he felt deep remorse.

> Down the years I have heard the cries of the dead in my dreams and in every waking moment. I will never be free of them. I have never been back there [to Auschwitz] because of my shame. This guilt will never leave me. I can only plead for forgiveness and pray for atonement.

And when he faced a judge earlier in the year, Gröning did not say that he was innocent because he was just a small cog in a gigantic machine. On the contrary, he openly admitted his guilt.

> It is without question that I am morally complicit in the murder of millions of Jews through my activities at Auschwitz. Before the victims, I also admit to this moral guilt here, with regret and humility.

What would Singer have told him? *Lighten up, man. Your net contribution to the death camp was zero. Get a life.* Why does this clash with our intuitions of moral responsibility? Why is it so repugnant? Because it is completely individualistic. He treats every human being simply as a faceless lump of humanity, not as a person linked to others by "the mystic chords of memory", kinship and shared experience. As a result, Singer's "effective altruism" has very little to do with what the rest of us understand by altruism. A superior term would be "effective bookkeeping".

The ultimate aim of Singer's book is to replace the most attractive feature of the Christian culture – its thousands of years of effective charity – with a different kind of do-good-ism. But it won't ever succeed because utilitarianism is about numbers. Christianity is about people.

Mr Spock, the comic utilitarian

MercatorNet, 6 March 2015

Why is there something faintly ridiculous in the logic of thinkers like Bentham, Mill and Peter Singer?

Mr Spock is dead. For the second time. This time for good. The actor Leonard Nimoy, who played the half-human, half-Vulcan in the cult classic TV series *Star Trek*, passed away this week at the age of 83.

His character died for the first time in *Star Trek II: The Wrath of Khan*, probably the best of the reboots of the TV series. In the concluding scene, the warp drive of USS Starship Enterprise has been damaged. Defying lethal doses of radiation, Spock enters the engine room, and restores power. In his dying moments, he speaks to Kirk through the glass doors.

> Spock: Don't grieve, Admiral. It's logical. The needs of the many outweigh ...
>
> Kirk: -- the needs of the few ...
>
> Spock: -- or the one... [He kneels.] I have been ...and always shall be ...your friend. [He places his hand on the chamber glass, and his voice is a whispered broken husk.] Live long and prosper!
>
> Kirk: [places his hand against the glass as Spock slumps and dies] No....

On the big screen, it doesn't sound so silly. Spock demonstrates in those few seconds the qualities which made him so memorable: unfailing loyalty to his fellow crew members, logic, lugubrious solemnity and utilitarianism. *The ways of the many outweigh the needs of the few* is a 23th century version of the slogan popularized by the 19th century philosopher Jeremy Bentham, *It is the greatest happiness of the greatest number that is the measure of right and wrong.* Isn't it amazing that it lasted all that time?

The writers of *Star Trek* enjoyed toying with philosophy and many episodes in the original series dealt with political or moral conundrums. There's a collection of essays on the ethics and metaphysics entitled *Star Trek and Philosophy: The Wrath of Kant*. And Georgetown University, in Washington DC, is offering a subject called "PHIL-180 Philosophy and Star Trek" this year. A focus on Mr Spock offers numerous chances to give utilitarianism a test drive.

With the possible exception of Peter Singer, Mr Spock of the pointy ears is the most famous utilitarian of our age. Which leads me to ask: why are utilitarian philosophers so often implausible human beings surrounded by a penumbra of absurdity?

First of all, Mr Spock. He is highly competent and supremely logical, but he fails to understand fundamental aspects of human experience. Take, for instance, his remarks about natural beauty:

> I've never stopped to look at clouds before. Or rainbows. You know, I can tell you exactly why one appears in the sky, but considering its beauty has always been out of the question. ("This side of paradise")

In other words, he is tone-deaf to a fundamental capacity of a rational person – aesthetic appreciation.

And Spock's bewilderment at romantic love often provides was grist for comedy. Dr McCoy sums up Spock's emotional barrenness:

> you'll never know the things that love can drive a man to... the ecstasies, the miseries, the broken rules, the desperate chances, the glorious failures, and the glorious victories. All of these things you'll never know,

simply because the word "love" isn't written into your book.

There's a bit of Dr Spock in all of the famous utilitarians.

Take Jeremy Bentham. He never married, had no children -- apart from Utilitarianism itself. He specified in his will that his body was to be preserved, dressed in his best clothes, and displayed in a glass cabinet to inspire "pilgrims [and] votaries of the greatest-happiness principle". He became a beacon of incandescent weirdness to light the paths of generations of utilitarians.

Take John Stuart Mill, the 19th century genius who popularized and softened utilitarianism. At the age of three he could speak both English and ancient Greek. By 12, he was devouring Aristotle's logic in the original. But when he was 20, he had a nervous breakdown, brought on by excessive ratiocination. He was a pleasant and urbane gentleman, but his romantic life was bizarre. At 24, although he was an eminently eligible bachelor, he fell in love with Harriet Taylor, a married woman. For 21 years, until her husband died, they carried on a deep and apparently chaste friendship, while living in a sort of *ménage a trois*. After they married, they had no children, although Mill was a devoted stepfather to Harriet's daughter.

Among our contemporaries, Peter Singer is the pre-eminent utilitarian. Like Mill, he is intelligent, urbane and deeply involved in public affairs. But as a logician, he even pips Mr Spock. Using his version of Bentham's "felicific calculus", he has constructed arguments justifying abortion, euthanasia, incest, bestiality and infanticide. Like other utilitarians he just follows the logic of his arguments wherever they lead. No doubt Singer is a thoroughly likeable and inoffensive fellow in private conversation, but he would unflinchingly argue for stewing babies in their mothers' milk if the argument took him there. Unlike Mr Spock, he is neither maladroit nor socially awkward. But like Mr Spock he seems perplexed by the emotional life. His conclusions are blood-curdling, but he is austerely detached from them. That's where the argument led me, he might say.

The same mephitic vapour surrounds lesser utilitarians, but it might be better not to name names. Beginning with the axioms of the felicific calculus, they reach bizarre conclusions by following the argument wherever it leads. Reducing the population by compulsory birth control. Using genetic engineering to reduce the average American height by 15cm to save energy. Reviving eugenics. Spiking the water supply with hormones to make people more moral. And many more story lines for future episodes of *Star Trek*.

In one of the most profound observations ever made about philosophy, Aristotle said "It was ... wonder, astonishment, that first led men to philosophize and still leads them." Dr Spock and his buddies philosophise using nothing but logic and, unsurprisingly, find nothing to wonder at; they live in the clouds instead of in the mire of human experience. Their inevitable pratfalls provide the perfect recipe for comedy.

Part 6

The reproductive revolution

The birth of Louise Brown, the first IVF baby, in 1978 marked the beginning of a new era for humanity. As Nobel laureate Robert Edwards recalled, "It was a fantastic achievement, but it was about more than infertility. It was also about issues like stem cells and the ethics of human conception. I wanted to find out exactly who was in charge, whether it was God himself or whether it was scientists in the laboratory." Ever since, the ethical problems have been multiplying. Nearly 40 years later, we have baby farms with surrogate mothers, embryos created and destroyed for research, half-animal, half-human embryos, gendercide and a host of other contentious issues. Who knows where it will end?

The controversial legacy of the father of IVF
MercatorNet, 16 April 2013

> *Robert Edwards, the inventor of IVF, died two days after Margaret Thatcher. History may show that his impact was even greater than hers.*

The creator of the first IVF baby, 2010 Nobel Laureate Robert Edwards, died last week. Obituaries and eulogies by colleagues, friends and admirers spoke of a passionate man with boundless energy, driven by a desire to bring happiness to infertile couples. Since he is directly responsible for the birth of some five million children since the first IVF baby in 1978, his legacy is worth pondering.

Like Margaret Thatcher, who was born in the same year and died two days before him, Edwards reshaped the world we live in. And as with Thatcher, we ought to ask whether it has been for the better.

Edwards was born in 1925 in Yorkshire. After a slow start in his research career, he began working in human reproduction in the mid-1950s. He teamed up with Dr Patrick Steptoe, an expert in the new field of laparoscopy in 1968. By 1969 they had provided the first compelling evidence that fertilisation could take place outside the human body. Characteristically, this development was announced on Valentine's Day.

At the time, the scientific establishment – to say nothing of the churches -- was strongly opposed. The reaction of the British Medical Association was so extreme that Edwards twice sued it for defamation. Eminent scientists described his work as immoral and criticised him as a self-publicist. James Watson, the Nobel laureate who discovered how DNA works, sneered at him. He lost government funding for his project.

Even the leading journal *Nature*, which backed his work, expressed some reservations. What was the point of bringing new children into an already over-populated world?

Fully aware that he was smashing as many idols as Thatcher did in political life, Edwards started to cobble together an ethical justification for his controversial research. In 1971 he wrote a paper (in conjunction with an American lawyer) for *Nature* on the ethics of IVF which anticipated many later developments.

Edwards was adept at public relations. He knew exactly what would happen once human reproduction became possible in laboratories and he tried to smooth a path for it. On the medical side he predicted sex selection, embryonic stem cell research, children for lesbians and single women, posthumous reproduction and genetic engineering. On the legal side he foresaw debates about over-population, gender imbalance, the personal identity of clones, and the need for government regulation.

When Louise Brown, a healthy 5 pounds, 12 ounces' baby, was born on July 25, 1978, criticism stopped. As Edwards triumphantly put it, "Most ethical disagreements have been vaporized" by the existence of millions of IVF babies.

What were the ethical principles which inspired him?

First, there should be no limits on scientific research as long as it does no harm. Science could not and should not be limited by ethics. As he told a journalist for the magazine *Living Marxism*, "I cannot accept this hyper-emotional stuff that says that some areas are out of bounds and cannot be touched."

In his hands, science was an attack upon the Christian world view. In 2003 he told the London *Times*: "[IVF] was a fantastic achievement, but it was about more than infertility. It was also about issues like stem cells and the ethics of human conception. I wanted to find out exactly who was in charge, whether it was God himself or whether it was scientists in the laboratory."

And what he discovered was that "It was us."

In principle nothing was out of bounds for scientists. His 1999 remarks backing eugenics are widely quoted: "Soon it will be a sin for parents to have a child that carries the heavy burden of genetic disease. We are entering a world where we have to consider the quality of our children." Edwards was actually in favour of human reproductive cloning, provided that the procedure was safe.

Second, the ethical norm for medicine (he was not a medical doctor) was the "clinical imperative". Whatever satisfies a patient's desires must be done. In 2004 he wrote: "Clinical imperative is a powerful doctrine, immediately accepted by many patients and professionals alike. A strong argument offered by many clinicians insists that any unwarranted restriction of scientific and clinical research must be rejected if it restricts the access of their patients to the most recent scientific advances."

This, obviously, can justify almost any medical procedure.

Third, human identify is proportionate to consciousness – which means that embryos, which have none, are just disposable organic material. Edwards was a fan of "practical ethics" – pragmatic justifications for his research. He wasted little time in debating issues like personhood. Why should he? They might have hampered his research.

As long as it undermined the humanity of the embryo, any reason, however specious, seems to have been good enough. One of his papers contains a bizarre passage drawn from evolutionary pantheism. "The broad evolutionary outlook [is] that life began only once and is continued as its spark is transmitted through successive generations via the gametes. Any decisions about the beginnings of human life will therefore be arbitrary and involve selecting a point where human life and dignity become paramount."

This is so silly that only an intellectual who has lost all faculty for self-criticism could propose it. If the beginning of human life is arbitrary, why not the end? Could we decree that life should end at 30, as in the film *Logan's Run*?

As with Mrs Thatcher – who, by the way, presided over the passage of the world's most liberal experimentation law in 1990 -- the fulsome praise heaped upon Edwards skips over some sticky questions, even for those who are not opposed to IVF.

Edwards's patients were not properly informed about the dangers of the procedure. (There were no animal trials for IVF (or for its successor, ICSI). Edwards did not seem to worry about the higher rate of birth defects among IVF children. They were just collateral damage of the "clinical imperative".

Feminists criticised Edwards for commodifying the female body. The magazine *Living Marxism* reminded Edwards of objections by the Feminist International Network of Resistance to Reproductive and Genetic Engineering. These women were arguing that IVF was "not invented to serve women's interests, but the needs and desires of medical scientists, and the state, to further technological progress and to aid population-control aims".

Edwards's response was apoplectic. "Look at the happiness of those women [his patients]," he said. "They wanted this treatment.

I am fighting for these women. Feminists should be arguing for more of this kind of help for women, not less of it."

Similarly, there is little discussion in Edwards's papers about the psychological welfare of the children created through IVF. What about the genetic orphans created through anonymous sperm donation? What about children of gay parents who will grow up without a mother or a father? More sad, but necessary, collateral damage.

The artificial reproduction created and defended by Edwards may someday be viewed as a technology more powerful than the atomic bomb. And perhaps like Edward Teller, the father of the bomb, another scientist without self-doubt, he believed that "There is no case where ignorance should be preferred to knowledge — especially if the knowledge is terrible". His blithe indifference to the social consequences of IVF is staggering.

Earlier this month an Australian bioethicist, Robert Sparrow, set out a blueprint for "in vitro eugenics" in the *Journal of Medical Ethics*. Generations of people can be created in Petri dishes, eliminating unsatisfactory genes in the quest for better human beings. Dr Sparrow calculates that two to three generations of human beings could be produced in a single year – rather than the 60 or so years that the pace of natural reproduction requires. "In effect," he writes, "scientists will be able to breed human beings with the same (or greater) degree of sophistication with which we currently breed plants and animals."

Is this chilling scenario the fault of the genial, baby-kissing professor who was Robert G. Edwards? It certainly is. There have been few scientists who envisaged the future more clearly and worked harder for it. "After such knowledge, what forgiveness?"

The dark past of anonymous sperm donation

MercatorNet, 25 January 2016

Few of the essentials have changed since the first recorded case in 1884

The use of assisted reproductive technology (ART) is so common nowadays that it's easy to forget how quickly social attitudes have changed. The Atlantic recently published a feature about the early days of artificial reproductive technology under the headline "The First Artificial Insemination Was an Ethical Nightmare: The 19th-century procedure involved lies, a secrecy pledge, and sperm from a surprise donor".

The implication is that that contemporary ART is far more ethical than it was in the bad old days. Is that true -- or has it just been dusted off and given a fresh coat of paint?

Let's look first at the origins of ART. The first pregnancy after artificial insemination apparently took place in England in 1790. The eminent surgeon John Hunter used the sperm of a "linen draper" to impregnate his wife. A doctor in France claimed that he had achieved eight successful pregnancies in the mid-1800s. An American doctor named Marion Sims attempted it several times in the 1860s with one pregnancy (which miscarried). He had to abandon his experiments after a public outcry.

All of these procedures involved the sperm of the husband. The first successful pregnancy after artificial insemination by donor was the topic of the article in The Atlantic. It took place in 1884 in Philadelphia but was not reported until 25 years later.

The patient was a married woman who had been unable to

conceive. After examining her thoroughly, the doctor, William Pancoast, realised that the problem probably lay with the husband. It turned out that he had become infertile after a bout of gonorrhoea which had happened before he was married.

Without seeking the consent of either husband or wife, the doctor anaesthetised the wife and inseminated her with the sperm of the best-looking of a small group of medical students, who were all sworn to secrecy. Pancoast eventually told the husband who, surprisingly, was delighted with the result. The woman never found out how she had become pregnant.

No report was made of this medical landmark until 1909. One of the medical students, Addison Davis Hard, by then a physician in Minnesota, published an account of the event in a medical journal. "That boy is now a business man of the city of New York and I have shaken hands with him within the past year," he wrote.

The main purpose of Dr Hard's contribution to the journal was to portray artificial insemination as a eugenic boon, "a race-uplifting procedure", which would generate children of "wonderful mental endowments" instead of "half-witted, evil-inclined, disease-disposed offspring". "Persons of the worst possible promise of good and health offspring are being lawfully united in marriage every day ... Artificial impregnation by carefully selected seed, will alone solve the problem."

In his opinion, a personal relationship with the biological father was of no importance whatsoever to the offspring: "The origin of the spermatozoa which generates the ovum is of no more importance than the personality of the finger which pulls the trigger of a gun ... It is gradually becoming well establisht [sic] that the mother is the complete builder of the child."

So there you have it: the whole ideology of assisted reproduction in one of its earliest defences -- the irrelevance of the institution of marriage, eugenics, the irrelevance of the father, faith in technology and trust in the integrity of the medical profession.

And one more thing. Who else could the father of this "business man of the city of New York" have been but Dr Hard himself? The pompous prose and the pseudo-scientific eugenic speculations cannot disguise 25 long years of yearning to hug that son he had so casually generated. ART cannot change human nature.

Has anything really changed since 1884? ART is increasingly divorced from marriage. Single women and lesbians shop for donors who will confer wonderful eugenic endowments upon their offspring. Many children become "genetic orphans" who will never know their fathers. To say nothing of the thousands of people who suffer the heartache of broken kinship links. Sperm donation always has been and always will be an ethical nightmare.

As a PS, the first significant article about artificial insemination by donor was published in the British Medical Journal in 1945. The authors, Austrian-born Bertold Wiesner and his wife Mary Barton and a colleague, described their experience at a London fertility clinic as a positive solution for male infertility. But many years later it emerged that Mr Wiesner himself was the father of perhaps two-thirds of the children produced at the clinic – probably about 600. No one knows how many because his wife had destroyed most of the records.

Donor insemination may blight the lives of children, but that's not the only evil. It also corrupts the character of the donors.

The Archbishop of Canterbury discovers his real father

MercatorNet, 11 April 2016

Shattering news about his paternity show how important biological roots are for all of us

In events which seem inspired by the script of a B-grade potboiler, the Archbishop of Canterbury, Justin Welby, the spiritual head of the world's Anglicans, has, at the age of 60, discovered that he is not who he thought he was.

After taking a DNA test to disprove rumours about his paternity, he learned that the rumours were true. His real father was the last private secretary of Winston Churchill, Sir Anthony Montague Browne.

His mother, Jane Gillian Portal, who also worked for Churchill, had a brief liaison with Sir Anthony, shortly before she eloped with Gavin Welby to the United States. She never suspected that her son Justin, who was born nine months after her wedding, was Sir Anthony's child. Her marriage to Welby was short-lived and she remarried in 1975, eventually becoming Lady Williams of Elvel. Welby died in 1977 of alcoholism.

Thanks to his deep religious faith, the Archbishop seems to have received the news with calm. He told *The Telegraph* (London) that "There is no existential crisis, and no resentment against anyone. My identity is founded in who I am in Christ."

He is obviously a strong and self-confident man who surmounted a difficult childhood with alcoholic parents to become a father of six children, a successful oil executive and then an Anglican priest. He had no idea that the ne'er-do-well whom he regarded as his estranged father was not. In a statement to the press he said:

> My own experience is typical of many people. To find that one's father is other than imagined is not unusual. To be the child of families with great difficulties in relationships, with substance abuse or other matters, is far too normal ...
>
> This revelation has, of course, been a surprise, but in my life and in our marriage Caroline and I have had far worse. I know that I find who I am in Jesus Christ, not in genetics, and my identity in him never changes ...
>
> At the very outset of my inauguration service three years ago, Evangeline Kanagasooriam, a young member of the Canterbury Cathedral congregation, said: 'We greet you in the name of Christ. Who are you, and why do you request entry?' To which I responded: 'I am Justin, a servant of Jesus Christ, and I come as one seeking the grace of God to travel with you in His service together.' What has changed? Nothing!

Although this extraordinary story is just an anecdote, it confirms what I've always thought should be one of the most important principles in contemporary bioethics: that every child deserves to know his or her biological parents.

Archbishop Welby was superbly prepared to survive a personal earthquake like this by virtue of his character and religious faith, but it was an earthquake nonetheless. That is perfectly understandable. People who discover late in life that they had been adopted are also deeply shaken.

To know who we are, to have a secure personal identity grounded in the facts of our biology, is an important dimension of our autonomy.

That's why Justin Welby's experience is relevant to the debate over the wisdom of same-sex marriage, a relationship which deprives a child of that connection with either a father or a mother. That intimate bond is not something which can be whisked away. It is a foundational part of our identity. Who knows what storms will rage in the hearts of children who learn as they grow up that their genetic parents had been deliberately excluded from their lives?

Oh well, people die

MercatorNet, 25 January 2011

A horrifying report from Philadelphia's district attorney will be abortion's Uncle Tom's Cabin.

First, sit down. If you are sitting down, take a deep breath. Because all this did not happen in a slum in Phnom Penh, or Sao Paulo, or Kinshasa. It happened in the United States, in Philadelphia, the birthplace of the nation. It happened only 100 miles from the guardian of the nation's freedoms, the *New York Times*.

This is about a charnel house which doubled as an abortion clinic for 30 years while regulators looked the other way.

This is about politicians in one of America's largest states who didn't want to rock the boat. This is about a cowardly bureaucracy in a city renowned for world-class doctors and hospitals. This is about doctors who refused to report one of their own.

This is about the betrayal of poor, scared women, mostly young, mostly black or immigrant. At least two of them are dead. Many had their wombs and bowels perforated. Many were infected with venereal disease with unsterilized instruments.

This is about hundreds of infanticides in which live, viable, babies in the third trimester of pregnancy were delivered – and then murdered by snipping their spinal cords with scissors. One of them was so developed that the doctor joked, before snipping, "he could walk me to the bus stop". It is about thousands of abortions.

"My comprehension of the English language doesn't and cannot adequately describe the barbaric nature of Dr Gosnell

The great human dignity heist

and the ghoulish manner in which he 'trained' the unlicensed, uneducated individuals who worked there," said the Philadelphia District Attorney, Seth Williams.

All this came to light on February 18 last year when the FBI and agents from the District Attorney's office raided the Women's Medical Society, on the corner of Lancaster and 38th Streets, in West Philadelphia. What they were seeking was evidence of illegal prescription drug activity by its director, Dr Kermit Gosnell. They found something far worse.

There was blood on the floor and urine was splattered on the walls. A flea-infested cat was prowling around, and there were cat faeces on the stairs. Semi-conscious women scheduled for abortions were moaning in the waiting room or the recovery room, where they sat on dirty recliners covered with blood-stained blankets.

The two surgical procedure rooms were filthy -- like "a bad gas station restroom", said a policeman. Instruments were not sterile. Equipment was rusty and outdated. Oxygen equipment was covered with dust. Corroded suction tubing for abortion procedures doubled as a suction source for resuscitation. It stank.

Foetal remains were haphazardly stored throughout the clinic – in bags, milk jugs, orange juice cartons, and even in cat-food containers. Some were in a refrigerator, others were frozen. The investigators found a row of jars containing just the severed feet of foetuses, like voodoo fetishes. In the basement, they discovered medical waste piled high.

Ambulances were summoned to pick up the waiting patients, but no one had the keys to the padlocked emergency exit.

Finally, after 31 years of abortion, infanticide, abuse, horror and murder, the doors of Philadephia's Women's Medical Society closed.

A Grand Jury investigated the Women's Medical Society last year. On January 19, its director, Dr Kermit Gosnell, and nine of his employees were indicted on various charges. The Grand Jury's 281-page report concluded: "Gosnell's 'medical practice' was not set up to treat or help patients. His aim was not to give women control over their bodies and their lives. He was not serving his community. Gosnell ran a criminal enterprise, motivated by greed."

Dr Gosnell appears to have earned between US$10,000 and $15,000 every night for a few hours of abortion work -- on top of illegally dispensing prescription drugs during the day. He has been charged with murdering one woman and seven infants, solicitation to commit murder, abuse of a corpse, corruption of minors, drug offenses, hindering prosecution, and violations of abortion law. His staff have also been charged with various crimes.

Dr Gosnell is probably on the road to jail. The district attorney may even ask for the death penalty.

But the Grand Jury report did not stop at cataloguing the horrors of the Women's Medical Society. It also pointed the finger at the supporting cast who chose to be silent while women were being butchered.

Two words sum this up. The Grand Jury cited a long list of moments stretching over decades when the state bureaucracy could have investigated complaints, could have intervened, could have inspected. A Nepalese immigrant, Karnamaya Mongar, even died after receiving too much anaesthetic at Gosnell's clinic as late as 2009, but no one acted. Why not? The chief counsel for the Pennsylvania Department of Health explained: "People die".

There was, says the Grand Jury report, a "complete regulatory collapse".

The Women's Medical Society was reviewed by state authorities when it opened in 1979. Ten years later it was reviewed again and numerous violations were found. Nothing was done. Reviews in 1992 and 1993 noted violations. Nothing was done. Then all reviews stopped. After the election of pro-choice Governor Tom Ridge (a Catholic, Republican, Harvard grad), "the Pennsylvania Department of Health abruptly decided, for political reasons, to stop inspecting abortion clinics at all".

Despite complaints from women injured by Dr Gosnell, despite complaints from a doctor about venereal disease transmission, despite a notification of an abortion of a 30-week-old baby carried by a 14-year-old girl, despite the death of Karnamaya Mongar, the Department did nothing.

Until the police raid and the publicity. Then they did something, all right. They hired lawyers to cover their butts in the coming investigation.

That was just the Department of Health. The agency which registers doctors and the agency which regulates public health also ignored complaints about the Women's Medical Society.

Then there were Dr Gosnell's colleagues. The world-renowned Hospital of the University of Pennsylvania is 20 minutes' walk away from the Women's Medical Society. A patient died at HUP after a botched abortion in 2000 and the hospital filed a report. But many of Gosnell's other victims were treated for abortion complications like perforated bowels and foetal parts in the uterus. Yet, says the Grand Jury report, "other than the one initial report, Penn could find not a single case in which it complied with its legal duty to alert authorities to the danger. Not even when a second woman turned up virtually dead."

Did "legitimate" abortion providers ring alarm bells? No. Dr Gosnell tried to join the National Abortion Federation in 2009. The evaluator rejected his application as the worst abortion clinic she had ever seen. But she told no one in authority.

The Grand Jury has summed up this conspiracy of silence in a single damning paragraph. "Bureaucratic inertia is not exactly news. We understand that. But we think this was something more. We think the reason no one acted is because the women in question were poor and of colour, because the victims were infants without identities, and because the subject was the political football of abortion."

There was "a blatant refusal to enforce the law" by the Department of Health. Why? The Department mentioned two reasons: the abortion providers might object and that abortion (which is legal in Pennsylvania up until 24 weeks) was "controversial". Such justifications, says the Grand Jury report, "are barely worth comment".

Are there other abortion mills like this in Pennsylvania? Its answer is dismaying: "We have no idea how many facilities like Gosnell's have remained out of sight, out of mind of DOH for decades – since they were first 'approved'." How many are there in other big American cities where bureaucracies which regulate abortion clinics are asleep at the wheel? In Boston, in Chicago, in Washington, in Houston, in Los Angeles, in San Diego? In New York?

Murders, abuse, bureaucratic cover-ups and negligence, a code of *omertà* among professional colleagues: isn't this red meat for crusading journalists? Apparently not. The *New York Times* – which crusaded so tenaciously last year about sex abuse -- yawned. A similar story in Bangkok received about the same amount of coverage last November: just a couple of stories buried in the back of the paper. What was displayed prominently was a revealing feature which appeared on January 21, the day after the abortion clinic story broke. It began: "Congratulations, New York City, did you hear the news? ... This is officially the abortion capital of America."

And two days after the story broke, President Obama re-affirmed his unconditional support for abortion: "today marks the 38th anniversary of Roe v. Wade, the Supreme Court decision that protects women's health and reproductive freedom, and affirms a fundamental principle: that government should not intrude on private family matters."

Isn't this evidence of the same wilful blindness as the bureaucrats in Philadelphia? No matter how appalling the news, abortion rights must not be questioned. No matter how many poor and ignorant girls and women are abused, abortion rights must continue.

What this case shows is that supporters of abortion rights are far, far, more interested in defending an ideology than protecting women. If Pennsylvania bureaucrats had done their job and intruded on "private family matters", a poor Nepalese refugee would be alive today.

As the Grand Jury Report put it, "We discovered that Pennsylvania's Department of Health has deliberately chosen not to enforce laws that should afford patients at abortion clinics the same safeguards and assurances of quality health care as patients of other medical service providers. Even nail salons in Pennsylvania are monitored more closely for client safety."

Abortion advocates contend that what women need is better regulation, not more restrictions. But what this horror demonstrates is that some regulators disdain their regulations. By shielding abortionists from the law, they have made the notion of safe and legal abortion a farce. In a just world, they should be charged with criminal irresponsibility.

In a final irony, America's leading centre for bioethics is located 10 minutes' walk from the Women's Medical Society at the University of Pennsylvania. Has the scandal on its doorstep rattled its bioethicists? Apparently not. The main article on its webpage advertises a new project on lesbian, gay, bisexual, transgender, queer, and intersex (LGBTQI) bioethics.

When will Americans wake up?

Designer babies? Don't leave it to bureaucrats to decide

The Age, 23 April 2002

The Hitchhiker's Guide to the Galaxy sheds some light on the reproductive revolution.

The late Douglas Adams, RIP, would have found a rich lode of material for one of his absurd novels in last week's news about IVF.

On Monday, a couple were given permission to create a designer baby to cure a youngster with anaemia. The Victorian Infertility Treatment Authority said this was ethical. On Tuesday, Monash IVF applied to screen embryos so that some couple's grandchildren would not have haemophilia in 30 years. Its ethics committee said this was ethical. On Thursday, a single woman was confirmed in her right to have IVF. All the relevant authorities said that this, too, was ethical.

I feel gobsmacked. It reminds me of the opening scene in *The Hitch Hiker's Guide to the Galaxy* when a Vogon spaceship announces that the planet is about to be annihilated.

> People of Earth, your attention, please. As you will no doubt be aware, plans for the redevelopment of personhood, family, and sexuality and morality require the building of a hyperspatial express route through your values, and regrettably they have been scheduled for demolition. An independent ethics committee has given its approval. The process will take slightly less than two of your Earth minutes. Thank you.

Don't we have a say? Or are we just supposed to collapse in terrorised acquiescence while terra firma boils away into space?

All the procedures approved last week in Victoria involve the destruction of human life and the creation of new parent-child relationships. All of us have a stake in whether these should be permitted. Even if you do not believe that the embryo is a human person, it is clearly human life.

French plans to bulldoze a World War I cemetery, disturbing the repose of Australian war dead, have caused a diplomatic ruckus. If we care this much for 90-year-old human skeletons, surely living embryos deserve respect as well?

But apart from the deeper philosophical and moral questions, who are these independent ethics committees wielding demolition beams at us earthlings? If last week is anything to go by, the role of ethics committees seems to be to approve everything that won't land you in jail. Instead of philosophers discussing life, the universe and everything, they are rubber-stamping bureaucrats who ensure that names are spelled correctly, boxes are filled in and the project is approved.

If ethics committees can authorise the extinction of human life, shouldn't their moral reasoning, procedural guidelines and financial interests be open to public scrutiny? At the moment, this is not happening. Indeed, it has been reported that the memberships of the two hospital ethics committees dealing with the "designer baby" case last week were kept secret, with Epworth and Monash Private Surgical hospitals refusing to comment on the case.

This lack of transparency is not only arrogant but alarming. It raises the suspicion that the principal ethic of ethics committees is to approve whatever employers want. What if this includes - as it soon will – sex selection, hybrid man-animals, or designer children?

And even if there are no financial incentives for institutional ethics committees to give the green light to their colleagues' experiments, there will be personal pressures. An MBBS or PhD is a warrant of intelligence, not impartiality or independent thinking.

The flurry of announcements last week underscores the urgent need for an independent review of Australia's institutional ethics committee system. This was the unanimous conclusion last year of the Kevin Andrew's federal parliamentary committee on cloning, which called for "greater transparency and accountability" in institutional ethics committees.

As the Queensland Bioethics Centre told the committee: "To leave oversight of this important area to such committees would do little to inspire confidence in the community that justice was being done, whatever the good intentions of individual committee members."

We don't pay taxes to live in a country run by doctors. The last country to experiment with medicocracy was the Serbian Republic of Bosnia under president Radovan Karadzic, a psychiatrist. That adventure had a very unhappy ending.

Debating diversity
Australasian Science, November/December 2009

Cheap diagnostic tests are on the way, but is Down syndrome the tip of the iceberg?

The Margaret River Burrowing Crayfish, the Orange-bellied Parrot, the Mountain Mistfrog and the Bare-rumped Sheathtail Bat are amongst 36 species listed by the Australian government as "critically endangered". If Dr Brian Skotko, of Children's Hospital Boston has his way, Down Syndrome children should be added to the list. In a recent issue of the journal *Archives of Diseases in Childhood* he points out that the number of DS children born is declining year by year, at least in developed nations.

Current studies show that 92% of women who receive a definitive prenatal diagnosis of DS choose to terminate their pregnancies. As a consequence DS children are vanishing. Because women are waiting longer before they have children and older women have a higher chance of having a DS child, the birth incidence should climb. In fact, it has actually decreased. For instance, in the US, without prenatal testing, there should have been a 34% increase in DS births, largely because of older mothers. Instead, there has been a 15% decrease – or a 49% gap. In the UK, there is a 48% gap. No doubt the statistics are similar in Australia.

And Skotko says that there will be even fewer of these children in the future because a non-invasive blood test will soon be available which will provide a definitive diagnosis in the first trimester. Two companies in the US have announced that they will market such a test later this year. Because it is uncomplicated, nearly all pregnant women will use it. Because it gives an early diagnosis, a woman will be able to terminate in the first trimester, so there will be less risk to her health. And because it is non-invasive, it poses no risk to the foetus before the diagnosis. Current tests entail a small risk of miscarriage, which means that sometimes a normal child dies in the course of testing whether it has Down Syndrome. In fact, a UK study last year claimed that for every 660 DS foetuses which are detected and terminated in each year, 400 normal children perish as well.

There will also be a financial incentive. Because the new tests are relatively cheap, health insurance plans will probably cover them, making their uptake even more widespread. DS children often have complicated health problems, and the insurers could see this as a cheaper option than paying for the medical care for the rest of their lives.

A plethora of knotty ethical problems are contained in this situation, even for those who accept a woman's right to choose an abortion. The obvious one is: what is really the big deal? "Parents who have children with Down Syndrome have already found much richness in life with an extra chromosome," writes Dr Skotko. Admittedly, DS children have impaired intellectual skills (although some have made it through university) but they are often extraordinarily loving, cheerful and affectionate. Parents often remark that they have special gifts that other children lack. What worries Skotko is that most doctors know very little about the positive side of life with DS and misrepresent the burden of raising a DS child. They often give inaccurate, incomplete and sometimes insensitive advice to women. He feels that this effectively makes it impossible for women to give informed consent.

The new non-invasive tests will make diagnosis of hundreds of genetic conditions possible before birth. DS is just the first of them. So in the not-too-distant future we are sure to debate what kinds of genetic variability we will tolerate in our society. An opinion piece in the leading journal *Nature* recently argued that "genetic diversity, from within or among groups, should be embraced and celebrated as one of humanity's chief assets". However, having drawn the line at DS, what other conditions will women be encouraged to terminate? Prenatal diagnosis is a mixed blessing: it gives knowledge, but not necessarily the ethical insight to use it wisely.

Marriage leads to children; gay marriage leads to surrogacy

Sydney Morning Herald, 19 July 2012

Cheap wombs might bring gay men the happiness of being the father ... but the cost of that happiness is often borne by poor and uneducated women

A TV show called *The New Normal* will have its premiere on NBC in the US soon. It's about a gay couple and the single mother they engage to have their baby.

"She's just like an easy-bake oven except with no legal rights to the cupcake," the surrogate-mother broker tells Bryan and David. This is a hard-nosed description of the woman's role in gay marriage and child-rearing, but it sums it up accurately.

In heterosexual relationships, the birth rate rises when couples are married. One would expect similar dynamics to apply to same-sex couples. For lesbian couples, this is not a huge problem; all they need is a sperm donor. But male couples need surrogate mothers.

Where will these women come from?

Unless the law of supply and demand is repealed, the answer is: where wombs are cheapest. At the moment, this is India, where surrogate motherhood has become a $2.3 billion industry, with the enthusiastic encouragement of some state governments. A recent investigation by the London *Sunday Telegraph* found there were only 100 surrogacies in Britain last year, but 1000 in India for British clients. The proportion in Australia is likely to be the same.

There are no official statistics, but it appears gay couples account for a substantial chunk of the overseas market. So will the legalisation of same-sex marriage lead to even more surrogate mothers in India? *BioEdge*, the bioethics newsletter I edit, emailed IVF clinics in India and the US asking whether they were preparing for a rising demand for surrogate mothers.

The answer was a resounding yes. Our survey is far from scientific, let alone comprehensive, but it suggests that poor women in developing or economically depressed countries will be recruited to service gay couples.

"The main reason patients travel from abroad to India is for excellent personal care, expertise and a lot of savings on the treatment costs," says Dr Samundi Sankari, of Srushti Fertility Research Centre in Chennai. "The costs that they pay here is almost one-fifth the costs they pay for surrogacy in US and Europe." He gets a lot of inquiries from gay couples in the US and Israel. Is he preparing for an increase in demand? "Definitely, yes."

Dr Samit Sekhar, of the Kiran Infertility Centre, in Hyderabad, also forecast an increase. He said a "sizeable number" of the centre's clients were gay. "We have seen an increase in the number of gay couples and single men approaching our clinic as soon as legitimacy to their public union is granted in their respective states or country."

There was one dissenting voice. A spokeswoman for Dr Shivani Sachdev Gour, of Surrogacy Centre India, Megan Sainsbury, was irritated. "We are not preparing for an expansion of services for gay couples. Why would you ask this?" However, most of the contented parents featured on Sachdev Gour's blog last month are gay.

Indian IVF clinics say surrogate mothers are adequately compensated. But it can be a dangerous job, and the contracts they sign are weighted heavily in favour of the commissioning parents. A surrogate mother in Ahmedabad collapsed and died in May, shortly before she was due. The client took the baby and her family was given only $18,000.

The award-winning British/Indian novelist and journalist Kishwar Desai deals with the surrogacy industry in her latest novel, *Origins of Love*. She told *The Guardian*: "There are hospitals where women are kept for the whole nine months while they carry someone else's child. There are good stories, where the surrogate is well looked after, but I would like to make people aware of the sheer exploitation of it, the fact that these women are extremely poor. They are carrying someone's child for two or three thousand pounds [$3000 to $4500]. They may do this three or four times. They may be forced to have a caesarean."

A leading US infertility doctor, Jeffrey Steinberg, who runs the Fertility Institutes in Las Vegas and Los Angeles, says he got a surge of inquiries whenever a jurisdiction legalised gay marriage. At the moment he uses only carefully screened American surrogates, but he is thinking of outsourcing their jobs to Mexico.

Supporters of same-sex marriage must recognise they face a serious moral dilemma. Cheap wombs might bring gay men the happiness of being the father of a child of their own. But the cost of that happiness is often borne by poor and uneducated women.

Part 7

Doctors at work

The great human dignity heist

Probably no profession is most trusted than health care workers. And with good reason: we place our lives in the hands of doctors. But many developments in modern bioethics are eroding that trust. Although doctors used to take the Hippocratic Oath to do no harm to patients, nowadays they can legally kill them in jurisdictions from Oregon to the Netherlands. Doctors are subject to the same temptations as the rest of us – greed, cowardice and ambition. If the boundaries are removed on protecting life at all costs, can the public still trust them?

Most medical research is wrong. I'm serious
Australasian Science, January/February 2011

An analysis of significant medical research papers has concluded that "most research findings are false for most research designs and for most fields".

Most of us have set pragmatism as our default position on bioethics. If it works, why not use it? If human embryonic stem cells are reported to be effective, for instance, what harm can there possibly be in using them? In fact, it may be immoral not to use them after the incredible progress reported in Nature!

But in an era of science by press release, pragmatists should know how reliable such reports are. And respected studies into the credibility of all medical research – not just on stem cells – suggest that claims of incredible advances are precisely that: incredible. In fact, according to a leading medical statistician, Greek academic John Ioannides, "most claimed research findings are false".

Dr Ioannides is not a crank or an enemy of science. On the contrary, his work has been published in leading journals and his claims are widely accepted among his colleagues. His groundbreaking 2005 paper in *PLoS Medicine* is the most downloaded in the journal's history. Every year he receives hundreds of invitations to speak at conferences. Doug Altman, the director of Oxford University's Centre for Statistics in Medicine, told *Atlantic*: "You can question some of the details of John's calculations, but it's hard to argue that the essential ideas aren't absolutely correct".

Ioannides' claims are largely statistical and thus require much brain cudgelling for laymen. But his conclusions ought to rattle anyone: that "most research findings are false for most research designs and for most fields" and "claimed research findings may often be simply accurate measures of the prevailing bias".

Why is this? There are a number of interlocking reasons.

Many studies are too small to be reliable. The best ones involve several thousand subjects but many studies, especially in genetics, are based on fewer than a hundred. Many studies are badly designed or are hard to compare with other studies of similar data.

Prejudice plays a role as well – although not necessarily ideological or financial. Scientists who are committed to a theory are less likely to find contradictory evidence. "Many otherwise seemingly independent, university-based studies may be conducted for no other reason than to give physicians and researchers qualifications for promotion or tenure," wrote Ioannides in his 2005 PLoS article. "Prestigious investigators may suppress via the peer review process the appearance and dissemination of findings that refute their findings, thus condemning their field to perpetuate false dogma."

Finally: "The hotter a scientific field (with more scientific teams involved), the less likely the research findings are to be true". Ioannides attributes this counter-intuitive effect to cut-throat competition to publish exciting research first. "This may explain why we occasionally see major excitement followed rapidly by severe disappointments in fields that draw wide attention," he says.

Isn't this relevant to far-reaching claims made for embryonic stem cells?

Even more discouraging for medical researchers is that the gold-standard of medical research, double-blind randomised trials, are not altogether reliable either. In another 2005 paper published in the *Journal of the American Medical Association*, Ioannides examined 49 of the top science papers of the previous 13 years. They had appeared in the best journals and had been cited extensively, yet between one-third and one-half of them were unreliable because they were later found to be wrong or exaggerated.

Although Ioannides' ideas are widely accepted, some researchers fear that they might be misinterpreted and used to debunk science or to promote shonky alternative therapies. He responds that truth is the best medicine: "The scientific enterprise is probably the most fantastic achievement in human history, but that doesn't mean we have a right to overstate what we're accomplishing".

Sound advice for the inner pragmatist!

I swear by Apollo, the healer (fingers crossed)

Australasian Science, June 2011

> *Doctors' attitudes to the Hippocratic Oath reveal that codes of conduct are not enough to produce ethical doctors – and scientists.*

Back in 2007, the UK's chief scientific advisor, Sir David King, published an ethical code for scientists. "Our social licence to operate as scientists needs to be founded on a continually renewed relationship of trust between scientists and society," he explained.

Since then the code has not had a lot of publicity. Perhaps this is the fate of pronouncements with which no one can possibly disagree. Who, after all, could quarrel with "Act with skill and care in all scientific work" or "Seek to discuss the issues that science raises for society"? "Minimise and justify any adverse effect your work may have on people, animals and the natural environment" is a bit more challenging, but any failure to minimise can always be offset by energetic self-justification. No one lobs nuclear missiles without some justification.

The model for the code was clearly the Hippocratic Oath, which was composed about 400 BC. Non-doctors commonly think that 25 centuries of the medical profession have been united in a solemn commitment to work for the welfare of their patients. It gives the medical profession an aura of integrity.

Surprisingly, though, the Hippocratic Oath is a relatively recent phenomenon. It was first administered to students at the University of Wittenberg in Germany in 1508. Not until 1804 in

France did it become a formal part of a graduation ceremony. And even in the 1920s in the United States only one-fifth of medical schools required it.

What made the oath popular was the disgraceful conduct of Nazi doctors who conducted barbaric experiments upon prisoners in jails and concentration camps. After World War II there was a movement to consciously reframe medicine as a humanitarian service rather than just as a technical discipline. This gave rise to codes of medical ethics, the emergence of bioethics and photos of medical students taking the Hippocratic Oath.

However, Hippocrates would not recognise his oath if he were to attend a graduation ceremony today. Obviously some of its anachronistic features had to go. Swearing by Apollo, Asclepius, Hygieia and Panacea is no longer binding. Hippocrates' students were exhorted to share their goods with their master and "To look upon his children as my own brothers". If only...

More controversially, the Greek oath contained clauses forbidding abortion and euthanasia. It was said to be the first time that killing and curing had been separated. Hippocrates was devoted only to healing his patients regardless of rank, age or sex. But both of these procedures are highly contested today. In a 1993 survey of medical oaths in the US and Canada, only 14% banned euthanasia, and only 8% abortion.

Hippocrates also took a much tougher line on sexual relations with patients. "In every house where I come I will enter only for the good of my patients, keeping myself far from all intentional ill-doing and all seduction and especially from the pleasures of love with women or with men, be they free or slaves." Only 3% of US and Canadian oaths prohibited such contact.

But the contemporary oath is more than window-dressing.

Physicians need to feel that their professional lives have a moral compass higher than self-interest. Furthermore, doctors know that regulations, financial incentives and public reporting are not enough to guarantee that patients receive the best possible care.

Updated oaths include clauses on issues like financial conflicts-of-interest, use of technology, medical error, whistle-blowing and racial discrimination. However, a survey in the Annals of Internal Medicine a few years ago indicated that doctors often ignore these guidelines. For instance, more than 90% agreed that doctors should report significantly impaired or incompetent colleagues – but only half did so.

A survey this year in the journal *BMJ Quality and Safety* found that only 80% of doctors strongly agreed that "Doctors should put patients' welfare above the doctor's own financial interests". About 8% did not agree that it was "never appropriate" to have a sexual relationship with a patient.

Perhaps the point is that protocols and codes are not enough to produce ethical doctors – and scientists. There has to be something deeper. Hippocrates would have called it virtue. But how to make people virtuous is a problem that we still are far from solving.

A deal with the devil after World War II
MercatorNet, 11 April 2014

Why did American officials refuse to prosecute Japanese doctors who had committed horrendous crimes in World War II

World War II is often called America's "good war" – a valiant struggle by a freedom loving democracy against vicious, racist, totalitarian tyrannies. There is much truth in this, but war is a dirty business and even from a good war it is hard to escape with clean hands.

One example of this which has come to light in recent years is the stomach-churning story of war crimes by Japanese doctors.

What happened in Nazi Germany is well-known. After the war, seven concentration camp doctors and officials were hanged and nine received severe prison sentences for performing experiments on an estimated 25,000 prisoners. Only about 1,200 died but many were maimed and psychologically scarred. Reflection on these crimes gave rise to the Nuremberg Code of medical ethics which spelled out doctors' responsibilities towards experimental subjects. This became the foundation of contemporary bioethics.

Every bit as grotesque and gratuitous were experiments performed by hundreds of Japanese medical personnel. In the infamous Unit 731 in Harbin, in northeastern China, an estimated 3,000 prisoners of war of many nationalities, including Chinese, Koreans, Russians, and Mongolians, died. In addition, tens, perhaps hundreds, of thousands of civilians died in epidemics after the Japanese field-tested germ warfare on them.

Many of the doctors had been sent to China from Japan's leading medical schools at the request of the Army. In return Unit 731 provided medical equipment and abundant opportunities for human experimentation. This has led one Japanese bioethicist to conclude that "the Japanese medical profession itself is guilty of the crime."

So what did the American occupation forces do to bring to justice the Japanese counterparts of the Nazi doctors?

Nothing.

Well, almost nothing. There was one small trial. In 1945 eight American airmen parachuted out of a disabled B-29 bomber over Japan. They were handed over to doctors at Kyushu University for vivisection and all of them died. After the war, 23 of the doctors were found guilty of various charges at a war crimes tribunal. But their sentences were later commuted and all were free again by 1958.

The atrocities in China, whose scale and horror dwarfed the fate of the unfortunate airmen, were ignored. The Soviet Union tried and found guilty 12 of the staff at Unit 731 in the 1949 Khabarovsk War Crime Trials. (Their sentences were remarkably light and all of them were repatriated in 1956.)

But American authorities were determined to cover up the crimes of Unit 731. They dismissed the trials as Soviet propaganda – which they were, of course, because the USSR wanted to embarrass the US. But the story which emerged from the Khabarovsk trials was basically accurate. However, it was not in America's interest to publicise it.

As a result, many of its doctors built successful careers in Japan after the War. The commander of the unit, Surgeon-General Shirō Ishii, lived out his days in relative obscurity. The man who succeeded him late in the war, Kitano Masaji, became head of one of Japan's leading pharmaceutical companies. Several directors of Japan's post-war National Institute of Health had been active participants in human experimentation during the 1930s and 1940s.

How could these men have possibly escaped justice when German doctors like Josef Mengele became by-words for unethical behaviour?

A fascinating answer to this question appeared recently in the *Cambridge Quarterly of Healthcare Ethics*. The facts are well documented, even if they are still not widely known.

To cut a long story short, American officials struck a deal with Shirō Ishii and his subordinates. They traded immunity from prosecution for access to information which had been gleaned from the ghastly Japanese experiments. In addition to biological warfare, these had included operations on Chinese prisoners without anaesthetic to practice surgical techniques under battlefield conditions, deliberately infecting prisoners with diseases, clinical trials of non-standard treatments, and testing human resistance to extreme conditions.

The US Army had been investigating biological warfare at Camp Detrick, in Maryland, but progress there was slow and the Japanese experience was quite "valuable". American scientists who had interviewed the staff of Unit 731 and examined their records were envious. They concluded that:

> Such information could not be obtained in our own laboratories because of scruples [sic] attached to human experimentation ... It is hoped that the individuals who voluntarily contributed this information will be spared embarrassment [ie, not tried for crimes against humanity] because of it and that every effort will be taken to prevent this information from falling into other hands [ie, the Soviets].

The remarkable feature of this investigation was this: it was not cynical diplomats or pragmatic soldiers who foiled attempts at prosecution; it was American scientists. It's one more example of how the quest for knowledge can subvert the moral scruples of highly intelligent men.

The scientists won over the US Army lawyers to their point of view. An Army task force concluded that, "The value to the US of Japanese [biological warfare] data is of such importance to national security as to far outweigh the value accruing from 'war crimes' prosecution." It was also highly cost-effective. Two scientists told the Army that Ishii's research had cost "many millions of dollars and years of work" and the US was effectively buying it for a "mere pittance".

From a distance of 70 years, what explains this moral blindness? How could the officials have ignored the need to redress the appalling injustices of ten years of horror, especially in view of the fact that their counterparts in Germany were putting Nazi doctors in the dock?

The article suggests two reasons. First, the Japanese military was so ruthless that it left no maimed survivors, no one to touch the hearts of newspaper readers, no wrenching stories of torment. Heart-stopping testimony from four Polish women who survived Ravensbrück concentration camp was powerful evidence at the Nazi doctors' trials. But all of the Japanese victims had been slaughtered. No one was left to display their scars.

Second, "wartime exigency". Many factors were at play: the American reluctance to antagonise the Japanese; the value of the information; keeping Soviet hands off the information. "Wartime exigency does more than simply prioritize national security over human rights," write the bioethicists. "It urges toughness and decisiveness in decision-making, such that a moral blindness that would be seen as a deficiency in other times is instead seen as a virtue and a necessity."

Several historians of these events have concluded that the American authorities were "accomplices after the fact" to the crimes of the Japanese doctors. Bioethicist Jing-Bao Nie has pointed out that Americans have little idea of the deep rage felt by the Chinese over what happened and subsequent Japanese denials. His proposal is that the US make an official apology and offer some compensation for this historical injustice. It seems like a good idea. Six decades of cover-up is long enough.

America's shame over syphilis experiments in Guatemala

Australasian Science, November 2011

President Obama's bioethics commission finds that US experiments in post-war Guatemala turned a blind eye to ethical concerns.

For the past year it has been bioethical bow, scrape and grovel time in Washington DC. After learning that American public health researchers had infected hundreds of Guatemalans with venereal diseases between 1946 and 1948, President Obama had to telephone his Guatemalan counterpart to apologise. He then set up a commission to investigate the appalling story of coercion and deception. A detailed historical report was published on 13 September.

The tale came to light long after the doctors and participants had passed away. After World War II, thousands of STD-infected servicemen were being demobbed. American public health officials needed to know more about the effectiveness of the new miracle drug penicillin to control the spread of STDs in the US, and after researching this on volunteers in an Indiana prison they went to Guatemala.

Dr John C. Cutler, a Public Health Service physician, first selected men in the Guatemala National Penitentiary, then men in an army barracks, and then men and women in the National Mental Health Hospital.

The commission concluded that researchers deliberately exposed about 1300 inmates, psychiatric patients, soldiers and commercial sex workers to syphilis, gonorrhoea or chancroid. Permissions were obtained from government authorities but not from individuals.

Initially the doctors used prostitutes with the disease to infect the prisoners (since sexual visits were allowed by law in Guatemalan prisons). When "normal exposure" failed to infect them they performed direct inoculations. These were made from syphilis bacteria poured onto the men's penises or on forearms and faces that had been slightly abraded. In some cases they used spinal punctures. The subjects were given penicillin after they contracted the illness.

The results were never published and gathered dust in archives at the University of Pittsburgh.

Even by the standards of the time, this project was regarded as unethical. After all, only a few months before, Nazi death camp doctors had been condemned to death and there were long prison terms handed out for medical experiments conducted without informed consent.

Principles later formalised as the Nuremberg code of medical ethics had been published in *the Journal of the American Medical Association* in 1947. In April 1947, New York Times science editor Waldemar Kaempffert observed, as if it were universally accepted, that deliberately injecting human subjects with syphilis microbes was "ethically impossible".

Despite this Cutler, who became a respected academic with an interest in population control, pushed ahead. "The attitude toward the Guatemalan people was pretty much what you'd expect if they were doing research on rabbits," said a member of Obama's commission, bioethicist John Arras of the University of Virginia.

Cutler's higher-ups in the public health hierarchy were more squeamish but they did not stop the project. His superior confided: "I am a bit, in fact more than a bit, leery of the experiment with the insane people. They cannot give consent, do not know what is going on, and if some goody organization got wind of the work they would raise a lot of smoke."

When the US Surgeon General, Thomas Parran, was told of the project he commented: "You know, we couldn't do such an experiment in this country". But he did not stop it.

Bioethics today tends to be more concerned with protocols than with judgmental words like "right" and "wrong". But President Obama's bioethics commission did not hesitate to describe the Guatemala experiments as "reprehensible" and "morally wrong".

The commission is currently working on a second report about standards for protecting human research participants. This is a live issue. Many pharmaceutical companies are outsourcing clinical trials to countries in the developing world where costs are lower and the paperwork is less onerous. There is enormous potential for the abuse of vulnerable people.

What lessons from this shameful episode can be applied to contemporary medical research?

One, says the commission, is "never to take ethics for granted, let alone confuse ethical principles with burdensome obstacles to be overcome or evaded". Another is that "the quest for scientific knowledge without regard to relevant ethical standards can blind researchers to the humanity of the people they enlist into research".

Eternal vigilance is the price of bioethical rectitude.

Part 8

Homo sapiens 2.0

The Time Machine, *the famous novel by the Victorian novelist H.G. Wells, envisages an age hundreds of thousands of years from now in which humanity has evolved into two species, the soft and pampered Eloi and the brutal and degenerate Morlochs. Some contemporary writers on bioethics foresee a future in which the world is divided between the gen-rich and the gen-poor, enhanced humans and ordinary humans. Developments in genetics and the reproductive revolution make this possible, if not probable. Are we ready for the moral challenges of a eugenic future?*

Engineering humanity

Australasian Science, July 2009

The Terminator movies raise the significant bioethical question of whether it is better to be a man or a machine.

Without Arnold Schwarzenegger, the fourth film in the series, *Terminator Salvation*, is a bit limp, in the opinion of most critics – notwithstanding the car chases, explosions, and high-tech shoot-outs. But, believe it or not, obscured by billowing clouds of smoke and spurts of flame, there is a significant bioethical question. Is it better to be a man or a machine?

Without revealing the absurdly convoluted plot, our saviour is a cybernetically-enhanced version of a prisoner executed in 2004. He wakes up in 2018 as a bewildered participant in a war between us and Skynet, an artificial intelligence system which has become conscious and turned on its creators. Most of humanity has been obliterated in a nuclear holocaust. Where do the loyalties of a half-human, half-machine cyborg lie? T4 has a heart and sacrifices himself to save humanity.

For most viewers, *Terminator Salvation* is as realistic as Goldilocks and the Three Bears. At least it has a sensible outcome: humanity wins.

But there are a number of computer experts whose hearts are with Skynet rather than the humans. They look forward to a future in which humanity will perfect itself by becoming more and more like super-intelligent machines. And they are already planning for its coming. They call it "the Singularity".

Ray Kurzweil, a legend in the IT world, a pioneer in optical character recognition, speech recognition and text-to-speech, has become the apostle of "the Singularity". This is the moment – it could happen by 2045 – when artificial intelligence becomes self-conscious and "alive".

This sounds nutty – "the Rapture of the geeks" is one unkind description – but if you remember Moore's Law, that IT capacity doubles every 18 months or so, it becomes slightly more plausible. Intelligent and well-heeled Silicon Valley residents, including Peter Thiel, the co-founder of PayPal, are enthusiastic supporters of the Singularity. Two films financed by Kurzweil are in production, *Transcendent Man* and *The Singularity is Near*.

Just one little question: what happens to us humans after 2045?

Well, the singularitarians have held three summits to discuss troubling issues like that. Perhaps we will be in charge of the machines; perhaps they will exterminate us, à la Skynet. The most exciting possibility is that we will be able to upload our brains onto computers and thus achieve a kind of disembodied cyber-immortality. This has generated some discussion about the ethics of copying and pirating intelligences.

So the question provoked by *Terminator Salvation* is this: is being plain old Humanity 1.0 worthwhile – in spite of our messy emotions, cloudy intelligence, imperfect bodies and unavoidable death? Or should we aspire to move forward to Humanity 2.0?

In fact, we are moving in the direction of Humanity 2.0, or "transhumanism", right now. Of course we are far away from immortality uploads. But living for a thousand years through strategies for "engineered negligible senescence" is a serious goal for some scientists. It even has its own journal, *Rejuvenation Research*.

Other scientists aspire to create "better humans" through genetic engineering. It is not yet possible – or legal – to created genetically enhanced children yet, but the time is not far off. Many IVF clinics already offer parents the possibility of sifting embryos for children who will not carry genes for certain genetic diseases. The next step is premier IVF to produce offspring with higher IQs or the bodies of super-athletes. Or both, if you can afford it.

As many bioethicists have noted, the notion of Humanity 2.0 opens a Pandora's box. If it becomes possible, society could end up divided between the gene-rich and the gene-poor. Mankind might eventually split into two distinct species, *Übermenschen* with an enhanced genome which confers longer life, freedom from disease, and freedom from violence -- and the rest of us *Untermenschen*.

This would spell an end to democracy and equality. That's why the well-known American political scientist Francis Fukuyama has called transhumanism "the world's most dangerous idea". "It is very possible, he writes, "that we will nibble at biotechnology's tempting offerings without realizing that they come at a frightful moral cost."

The point is that the dilemma faced by the saviour cyborg is one that we will face in real life in the not-too-distant future. Should we seek to become better humans by modifying ourselves with technology or in the old-fashioned way, with politics and moral codes? *Terminator Salvation* may offer mindless violence, but it is not altogether brainless.

Seeking eternal life in a freezer

MercatorNet, 17 September 2015

> *Kim Suozzi, the young American woman with cancer who froze her head.*

What would the 17th century French mathematician and philosopher Blaise Pascal think of cryonics -- the business of freezing people until scientists can revive them? Given his sceptical turn of mind and his religious fervour, not much. However, a few years ago David Shaw, a Scottish bioethicist, thawed out Pascal's famous wager to defend it.

Some readers might recall that Pascal's Wager works like this. If you are a betting man, he argued, it is preferable to put your chips on the existence of God because the benefits of the afterlife are so great that they dwarf the fleeting pleasures of atheism. As theology, Shaw says, this argument has been discredited. But it does succeed for cryonics:

> At worst, cryonics offers a slim chance of living for a few more years. At best, it offers a slim chance of living forever. Ultimately, the Cryonic Wager is overwhelmingly attractive for the rational humanist, even without the prospect of eternal life.

It makes sense, Shaw argued, because "for atheists who don't believe in an afterlife, cryonics represents the only chance of life after 'death'".

Alcor, an American company in Scottsdale, Arizona, which freezes whole bodies (US$200,000) and neuropatients (ie, heads, $80,000) and the occasional cat or dog, is the best-known practitioner of cryonics. It currently has over a thousand members enrolled and about 140 patients in its freezers. As soon as a member is pronounced clinically dead, its doctors jump into action, place the patient in a ventilator and begin the freezing process.

While this may sound quite weird, cryonics and other life extension technologies have captured the imagination of some of the brightest minds in Silicon Valley. There's a certain life-cycle symmetry to it: if embryos can be frozen and revived, why can't adults?

Part of Google's recent reorganisation involved the creation of a spin-off company, Calico, which does research into longevity. Peter Thiel, the billionaire venture capitalist and co-founder of PayPal, has made substantial investments into a foundation called Strategies for Engineered Negligible Senescence. Thiel has also signed up with Alcor.

The *New York Times* recently highlighted the case of one of Alcor's "patients", 23-year-old Kim Suozzi, who died of brain tumour in 2012. She crowd-financed the preservation of her head (a process euphemistically called "cephalic isolation") on Reddit.

A head might not seem very useful without a body, but the theoreticians of cryonics believe that someday it will be possible to make a digital copy of the brain's wiring, called a "connectome". This would be uploaded to a computer and hooked up to sensory devices. Someday, it may be possible to power a robot with Kim's connectome. Someday, she may live again.

That "someday" may be a long time in coming. If the connectome for a human brain is every mapped, it could be as large as 1.3 billion terabytes, which is not something you can carry around on a memory stick. In fact, the collective capacity of the world's hard drives is an estimated 2.6 billion terabytes.

A number of interesting ethical questions are provoked by cryonics. Is the self the connectome? Is the body part of the self? Is Alcor cheating its patients (ie, customers)? Is it better to spend the freezing fees on charity? Is it moral to extend the lives of rich who can afford cryopreservation?

But the central issue is whether immortality is a good thing. The aspiring immortals in Silicon Valley don't plan to succumb to the ravages of old age, or to wake up in a diminished state. But the wisdom of the ages, from the Bible and the Greeks to modern times, is that you can have too much of a good thing.

In *Gulliver's Travels* there is an unsettling description of the immortal "struldbugs" on the island of Luggnagg – immortal, but not young and not healthy. "They were the most mortifying sight I ever beheld; and the women more horrible than the men," says Gulliver. "Besides the usual deformities in extreme old age, they acquired an additional ghastliness, in proportion to their number of years, which is not to be described."

Cryonics faces a significant consumer resistance because of the "Yuck" factor – after more than 40 years and steady publicity, Alcor still has only a few score patients. When Kim disclosed her plan to her father, he said "I can't help you with this. We don't live forever, Kim." Most people, religious or not, would agree with him.

What accounts for that instinctive feeling?

Death is never welcome, but perhaps we fear immortality too. The human mind, let alone the body, is not fashioned for unending cycles of experience. After a few hundred years, even Methuselah must have been itching with boredom. The great 19th century English poet Tennyson reworked the ancient Greek legend of Tithonus, a young man who asked his lover, the goddess Aurora, for immortality. He ends like the Struldbuggs and envying "the homes / Of happy men that have the power to die, And grassy barrows of the happier dead."

Perhaps it is better to see life as a limited-overs competition to do the best job we possibly can before we are bowled out.

What if computers have feelings, too?
Australasian Science, July/August 2014

> *If software becomes intelligent, what are the ethics of creating, modifying and deleting it from our hard drives?*

Most bioethical discourse deals with tangible, nitty-gritty situations like surrogate mothers, stem cells, abortion, assisted suicide, or palliative care. After all, the "bio" in bioethics comes from the Greek word *Bios*, meaning corporeal life. Historically the field has dealt with the ethical dilemmas of dealing with blood and guts.

But there is a theoretical *avant garde* in bioethics, too. It's a bit more like science fiction than ER. Theoretical bioethics tries to anticipate ethical issues which *could* arise *if* advanced technology becomes available. There are always a lot of ifs – but these are what bring joy to an academic's heart.

The other day an intriguing example lobbed into my in-box. Writing in the *Journal of Experimental & Theoretical Artificial Intelligence*, Oxford bioethicist Anders Sandberg asks whether software can suffer. If so, what are the ethics of creating, modifying and deleting it from our hard drives?

We're all familiar with software that makes *us* suffer because of corrupted files and crashes. But whimpering, yelping, whingeing software?

This is a bit more plausible that it sounds at first. There are at least two massive "brain mapping" projects under way. The US$1.6 billion Human Brain Project funded by the European Commission is being compared to the Large Hadron Collider in its importance. The United States has launched its own US$100 million brain mapping initiative. The idea of both projects is to build a computer model of the brain, doing for our grey matter what the Human Genome Project did for genetics.

Theoretically, the knowledge gained from these projects could be used to emulate the brains of animals and humans. No one knows whether this is possible, but it is tantalising for scientists who are seeking a low-cost way to conduct animal experiments.

As one theorist has written: "the first machines satisfying a minimally sufficient set of constraints for conscious experience could be just like ... mentally retarded infants. They would suffer from all kinds of functional and representational deficits too. But they would now also subjectively experience those deficits."

This implies that a being – is it too much to call it a person? — is alive on the hard drive. And building on the ethics of animal experimentation, it could be argued that tweaking the software to emulate pain would be wrong.

How would we know whether the software is suffering? That is a philosophical conundrum. Sandberg believes that the best option is to "assume that any emulated system could have the same mental properties as the original system and treat it correspondingly". In other words, software brains should be treated with the same respect as the experimental animal; virtual mistreatment would be just as wrong as real mistreatment in a laboratory.

How about the most difficult of all bioethical issues, euthanasia? For animals, death is death. But if there are identical copies of the software, is the emulated being really dead? On the other hand, would we be respecting the software's dignity if we kept deleting copies?

Even trickier problems crop up with emulations of the human

brain. What if a virus turns software schizophrenic or anorexic? "If we are ethically forbidden from pulling the plug of a counterpart biological human," writes Sandberg, "we are forbidden from doing the same to the emulation. This might lead to a situation where we have a large number of emulation 'patients' requiring significant resources, yet not contributing anything to refining the technology nor having any realistic chance of a 'cure'."

And what about software "rights"? Could the emulations demand a right to be run from time to time? How will their privacy rights be protected? What legal redress will they have if they are hacked?

The imaginative dilemmas projected by Sandberg and his fellow futurists cannot be falsified because they haven't happened yet. My bet is that they will never happen. But there is a take-away. If human beings are not unique and if our respect for beings is proportional to their consciousness, then we stumble into huge (and unnecessary) dilemmas. Radical animal rights activists claim not only that primates and dogs should not be experimented upon, but also animals with less consciousness like mice. Any being that can suffer deserves protection and respect.

The same reasoning leads, as Sandberg demonstrates, to the notion of suffering software and enforceable rights for software. It is this *reductio ad absurdum* which ought to make us question whether we have properly understood the notion of "animal rights".

Part 9

Grey matter

The brain is the outer space of inner space, a mysterious, hardly explored galaxy within us. Governments are pouring hundreds of millions of dollars into neuroscience research, hoping to find the key to curing degenerative conditions like Alzheimer's and Parkinson's disease. But defence planners and business are also interested, as unlocking the secrets of the brain could lead ways to influence and even manipulate human behaviour. There is no end to the ethical complications that scientists will face.

Are amnesia drugs on the way?
Australasian Science, April 2009

There is enormous commercial potential for a drug which can erase bad memories.

In the film *Eternal Sunshine of the Spotless Mind*, Jim Carrey and Kate Winslet use a specialist medical service to obliterate their memories of their relationship. Science fiction? Only for the time being, it seems. The Dutch authors of a recent study in *Nature Neuroscience* think that they are on track to developing a drug to blunt bad memories. The practical applications are immense. A spotless mind pill could bring relief to millions who suffer from post-traumatic stress disorder.

Here's what the researchers found. When 60 student volunteers saw pictures of spiders they received a mild electric shock, enough to develop a fear response. Then half of them received the beta-blocker propranolol, a drug used to steady the heartbeat; the control group only a placebo. The students who received propanolol were able to look at the spiders without fear. In other words, their emotional memory had been erased, but not the declarative memory of the spider images themselves.

This is consistent with previous research which suggests that emotional memory is controlled by the amygdala in the brain and declarative memory by the hippocampus. Perhaps propanolol disrupts protein synthesis in the amygdala, the researchers hypothesised.

How significant is this particular study? Not very, in all likelihood, despite lurid tabloid headlines. "All they've shown so far is that the increased ability to startle someone if they are feeling a bit anxious is reduced," says Professor Neil Burgess, of the Institute of Cognitive Neuroscience, in the UK.

However, it is a harbinger of the future with far-reaching bioethical implications. The US President's Council for Bioethics devoted a whole chapter to an ethical analysis of memory-blunting in a recent white paper on biotechnology. "Although the pharmacology of memory alteration is a science still in its infancy, the significance of this potential new power... should not be underestimated," it said.

There is enormous medical – and commercial – potential for a successful drug. A recent Pentagon study has estimated that 11 percent of Iraq veterans and 20 per cent of Afghanistan veteran suffer from post-traumatic stress disorder – perhaps 300,000 people. Currently the problems of PTSD sufferers in the military range from simple readjustment to suicide and murder. A drug would allow soldiers to retain declarative memories of injury and death without their incapacitating emotional intensity.

But even using memory-erasing drugs in combat is ethically ambiguous. We are only at the threshold of understanding how memory is integrated into our personal identity. Blunting the memory of trauma might bring short-term benefits but long-term anxiety. And what about legitimate feelings of guilt and shame? These drugs could be used to numb the consciences of soldiers so that they would kill without remorse.

"One of the horrible things I discovered after the [first] Gulf War was that, because of the coeducation of wars, as it were, male soldiers were given extensive desensitization training to make them able to hear women being raped and tortured in the next room without breaking," the former chairman of the US Bioethics Council, Dr Leon Kass, has said. "It's a deformation of the soul of the first order. I cannot speak about it without outrage."

If they fell into the wrong hands, memory-blunting drugs could be used by abusers to soothe victims by removing their resentment and anger. Sharon Begley, of *Newsweek*, saw flashing lights ahead after the release of the Dutch study: "let's face it, given the slippery slope of drug use, it will be a short step from erasing the memory of a brutal rape or a roadside bomb in Iraq to erasing the memory of a bad date".

Furthermore, as a community we feel that some painful memories should never be forgotten. Should survivors of the Rwandan genocide have been given propranolol or should they demand justice for the crimes they suffered? Part of being human is learning from the painful memories of catastrophe.

While memory-blunting drugs have enormous potential for treating patients with emotional disorders, their use will have to be carefully controlled. They could have unpredictable effects. After all, the treatment given to Carrey and Winslet worked so well that they fell in love all over again. Those who ignore their memories are destined to repeat them.

If you're not a criminal, you've got nothing to worry about

Australasian Science, June 2010

When the DNA profiles of innocent people are kept by law enforcement agencies it places them at risk of a lifetime of genetic surveillance.

One of the longest-running TV shows in the US is *America's Most Wanted*, a reality show that gets viewers to dob in murderers, rapists and child molesters. To date, it claims to have fingered 1110 criminals.

Such is its popularity that in March host John Walsh celebrated the 1000th episode at the White House. President Obama used to be a law lecturer, but it didn't take much arm-twisting to get his personal backing to taking and retaining DNA samples from individuals arrested for a crime but not convicted. "No different than fingerprinting or a booking photo," said Walsh, and Obama nodded sagely and replied: "It's the right thing to do".

But is it? Experts on human rights say no.

The European Court of Human Rights may have slowed down Britain's rapid move to almost-universal DNA profiling. In a 2008 judgement it found that indefinite retention of DNA samples from everyone who is arrested, regardless of their age or guilt, was a violation of a basic right to privacy.

The database in the UK includes more than five million DNA profiles, and one-fifth of these come from people without a criminal record. However, the government has been reluctant to destroy profiles because police and the public feel that DNA records are vital to putting criminals behind bars. The argument is that if you're not a crim, you've got nothing to worry about.

Apart from privacy concerns, many experts worry that the technology for forensic investigation is far from perfect. Here in Australia, Victorian police were forced to suspend the use of DNA evidence for a month last year after a substantial miscarriage of justice. A 20-year-old, Fara Jama, spent 18 months in jail for a rape he didn't commit. It turned out that DNA taken from him 24 hours before the crime over an unrelated offence for which he had not even been charged had contaminated the crime scene evidence.

How could that ever happen? Lawyers attribute it to the "white coat syndrome" – the power of shuffling statistics and graphs and figures before a mesmerised audience. Colin Powell did it to the United Nations when he used high-resolution images to "prove" that Saddam Hussein had weapons of mass destruction. And ordinary juries are no less susceptible to the allure of exact numbers and scientific precision.

A recent study by the Australian Institute of Criminology reported that juries are 23 times more likely to bring in a guilty verdict in murder cases if there is DNA evidence, and 33 times more likely in rape cases. There is a lot of concern that jurors, in the words of one judge, can be "overawed by the scientific garb in which the evidence is presented, and attach greater weight to it than it is capable of bearing".

Like mathematics, science is logical. But unlike mathematics, the results of scientific work have to be filtered through instruments and technicians and interpreted by experts. There is abundant room for unexpected error.

Erin Murphy, a legal academic at Berkeley, summed up

concerns in a recent article: "Even DNA typing – the archetypal objective science – requires an analyst to make judgment calls separating signal from noise. Just because a discipline is founded in scientific principle does not mean that it always yields wholly determinate answers: there is meteorology and there is math."

In fact, as pointed out recently in the *Los Angeles Times* by Osagie K. Obasogie of the Center for Genetics and Society in California, DNA testing is still an art as much as a science. Even though everyone's DNA is unique, current tests still have a surprising margin for error. "The entire enterprise of DNA databases is based on the idea that no two people share the same profile. But Arizona's database of 65,000-plus entries was shown to have more than 100 profiles that were similar enough for many experts to consider them a 'match'," he wrote.

Over-reliance on DNA profiles in crime investigation is just one facet of a growing acceptance of genetic determinism – the assumption that we are our DNA. More sophisticated techniques and protocols may eventually iron out the wrinkles with forensic evidence. But we can expect other important human rights debates as governments come to rely more and more upon genetic profiling for health care delivery, identification and security systems.

President Obama was extremely unwise to endorse a government database that could place citizens at risk of a lifetime of genetic surveillance.

Anti-Love Potions
Australasian Science, January/February 2014

What are the potential uses and consequences of a pill that could make people fall out of love?

The British novelist and playwright Somerset Maugham (1874-1965) has never faded away. His 1925 novel *The Painted Veil* was made into a film only a couple of years ago for the third time.

What I liked when I first read his stories was the geometric precision of his plots and his Edwardian gift for epigrams. "She plunged into a sea of platitudes, and with the powerful breast stroke of a channel swimmer made her confident way towards the white cliffs of the obvious." If only I could write like that!

But he had the misfortune of immense popularity and the critics have not been kind to him.

What I liked less and less as I grew older was his brutal cynicism. Much of that must be attributed to a tormented emotional life: a very unhappy childhood, a very unhappy marriage, and a succession of gay lovers. He used an early affair as the basis for his 1915 novel *Of Human Bondage*. This dealt with Philip Carey, a young doctor, and his senseless and unrequited passion for a Cockney waitress: "He did not care if she was heartless, vicious and vulgar, stupid and grasping, he loved her." The novel must have struck a chord, as three films have been based on it.

Here was a man, if ever there was one, made for the "anti-love biotechnology" discussed by bioethicists from Oxford University, including Julian Savulescu, in a recent issue of the

American Journal of Bioethics.

What if you wanted to fall out of love, as Maugham's hero did? You could simply take a pill and the passion would vanish. Of course, this is largely conjecture. The closest treatment at the moment is chemical castration for paedophiles and rapists, and that would be unlikely to interest Philip Carey, or anyone else, for that matter.

Nonetheless, there have been promising developments and Savulescu et al believe that we should work out the ethical issues as soon as possible.

A pill could be useful, they say, in a number of situations, including adulterous love, suicidal love, incestuous love (not that all incest is bad, they hasten to add), paedophilia, or love for a cult leader.

But a woman who can't find the strength to leave an abusive and violent partner is the clearest candidate for a break-up pill. They set four conditions for its use:

- The love must be clearly harmful;
- The person must be willing to use the pill;
- The pill would help a person follow higher order goals instead of lower order feelings;
- There is no other alternative.

They conclude that: "the individual, voluntary use of anti-love biotechnology (under the right sort of conditions) could be justified or even morally required. That is, in some cases, to deny its use would be inhumane."

There is one bitterly contentious issue, of course. What about homosexuality? In a sense, "reparative therapy", or helping gays to turn straight, is a primitive kind of break-up pill – but many people condemn this.

Savulescu et al make no exception for homosexual feelings. We must "also respect the autonomous decision of each individual to engage in her own process of 'becoming' who and what she seeks to be, in accordance with her personal goals and values," they argue. "Therefore, we must conclude that even in the controversial case of homosexual love, it may be possible to justify the use of anti-love biotechnology in certain cases."

I'm sceptical about the effectiveness of modern love potions. There are social and psychological components to addiction, for instance, which may be just as important as physiology. If we don't understand drug addiction, can we ever reduce love to "a suite of neurochemical and behavioural subsystems that evolved to promote the reproductive success of our ancestors"?

Fanning the smouldering fires of lust might be easier, but this will lead to horrendous abuses. People could spike drinks for one-night stands, quench teen romances, manipulate matchmaking, turn gays straight, turn straights gay... The ethical dangers are immense.

"The imminent development and availability of pro-love and anti-love agents will present a serious risk for unethical attempts to surreptitiously manipulate emotional and romantic feelings," commented two academics from Arizona State University.

And what if armies used it to suppress humane feeling to make soldiers crueller, more unforgiving, more full of hatred? Less sophisticated versions of this hypothetical drug were used effectively in the Liberian civil war -- which is why so many civilians there are missing hands, arms and legs.

Anti-love biotechnology could make a great script for a film -- but it will be *The Hangover IV* rather than *Of Human Bondage IV*. I wonder if we should treat it more like a banned chemical weapon rather than a medicine.

The larger question is whether relying upon technology instead of upon our intellect and will to master our emotions leads to human flourishing. What if we really could turn the well-springs of Eros on and off like a tap? It would be a great loss if a future Somerset Maugham were to solve his personal dramas with a pill so that he could lead a humdrum life as a suburban GP. As John Stuart Mill said, "It is better to be a human dissatisfied than a pig satisfied".

How about an "immorality pill"?

Australasian Science, May 2012

> *If a morality pill can induce moral behaviour, what could governments do with an "immorality pill" to control its citizens, law enforcers and soldiers?*

Not long ago, Princeton bioethicist Peter Singer, together with research assistant Agata Sagan, proposed a "morality pill" in a column in the *New York Times*. They speculated that moral behaviour is at least in part biochemically determined, so why not engineer moral behaviour with drugs? Here is the scenario that they painted:

> If continuing brain research does in fact show biochemical differences between the brains of those who help others and the brains of those who do not, could this lead to a 'morality pill' – a drug that makes us more likely to help? Given the many other studies linking biochemical conditions to mood and behaviour, and the proliferation of drugs to modify them that have followed, the idea is not far-fetched. If so, would people choose to take it?

This is not an altogether novel idea for Australian philosophers. Julian Savulescu, Peter Singer's one-time student, is even more radical. A couple of years ago he and Ingmar Persson contended:

> If safe moral enhancements are ever developed, there are strong reasons to believe that their use should be obligatory, like education or fluoride in the water, since those who should take them are least likely to be inclined to use them. That is, safe, effective moral enhancement would be compulsory.

Predictably, the proposal provoked a number of comic

responses — women don't need a morality pill, men do; we should have given one to Bush and Cheney; would it work on Wall Street, and so on. But it's obviously a serious proposal, so it needs to be taken seriously.

First of all, would it work? Humans have been experimenting with mood modulators for centuries, but all of them have problems. Alcohol is addictive; tobacco is carcinogenic; ecstasy can make people suicidal. There could be unpredictable and unpleasant side-effects. Would a morality pill with a morning orange juice really turn everyone into Mother Teresa?

Second, who defines what is moral? The governors of *Brave New World* decreed that moral behaviour meant being placid, happy and law-abiding, so they encouraged the inhabitants to dose themselves with soma. Will the government ideal be the gentle pacifism of Buddha or the warrior ethic of Nietzsche? What would stop governments from creating a pill to make soldiers pitiless, cunning and cruel?

Third, the morality in a pill might be all but indistinguishable from harsh social control. It could be a very attractive option for governments who want docile citizens. In fact, law enforcement officials have often turned to the medicine cabinet to make people moral. In several countries and in some American states, sex offenders have the option of chemical castration with anti-libidinal drugs. Soviet psychiatrists used drugs to cure dissidents of the illness of political deviations.

Fourth, the larger philosophical issue is whether it would be moral to distribute morality pills. The pills would reduce our autonomy and free will, which most people regard as a good part of what makes us human. If pills simply suppress impulses to participate in antisocial behaviour, are they really making people more moral or are they simply imposing mind-forged manacles on our freedom? Singer and Sagan anticipate this objection, of course, but they get around it by denying the existence of free will.

The promise of chemically induced bliss as a way of reducing social problems has bewitched writers from Homer (the lotus-eaters) to Timothy Leary (LSD). With the explosion of neuroscience, we can expect many more proposals like this.

But with respect – for Singer is said to be the world's most influential living philosopher and Savulescu is an Oxford don – I am more than a bit sceptical.

No job for addicts
Australasian Science, March 2013

Neurosurgeons in China are treating drug addicts by destroying a part of the brain responsible for feeling pleasure.

Chinese neurosurgeons are treating heroin addicts by destroying a region of the brain which feels pleasure. But, reports Time magazine, this "risks permanently ending the entire spectrum of natural longings and emotions, including the ability to feel joy."

Even in China, zapping bits of the brain is controversial. The Ministry of Health banned it in 2004 – but left a loophole for researchers. Apparently one surgeon drove a truck through this loophole and by 2007 he had done 1,000 of these operations to treat severe depression, epilepsy and schizophrenia.

And it is still happening. In October, doctors at Tangdu Hospital at the Fourth Military Medical University in the city of Xi'an, reported the results of neurosurgery on drug addicts -- ablation of the nucleus accumbens -- in a major international journal, *World Neurosurgery*.

They found that it was effective in getting addicts off drugs, but only in about 58% of them – compared to a 30-40% non-relapse rate for conventional treatments. There are also side-effects, although the doctors say that these are relatively minor. For such a drastic treatment, then, the odds of success are quite low.

Time cited a number of ethical concerns. First, animal studies suggest that the ablation of the nucleus accumbens did not stop the craving for opioids. Second, there may be a lack of informed consent. Drug addiction is a capital crime in China and patients may be clutching at straws to stay out of the courts. Third, publishing the results of unethical research may itself be unethical.

Fourth, the risks seen to outweigh the benefits. While the operation might be acceptable for long-term addicts, a recent article mentioned that some patients were only 19 and had been addicts for only 3 years. "Addiction research strongly suggests that such patients are likely to recover even without treatment, making the risk-benefit ratio clearly unacceptable."

So from a consequentialist standpoint, the numbers do not add up for ablation of the nucleus accumbens. But imagine for a moment that the Chinese scientists were ethically irreproachable. If that were the case, my guess is that Western neurosurgeons would be quite interested. In fact, the Portuguese neurosurgeon Egas Moniz won the 1949 Nobel Prize for Medicine for developing the frontal lobotomy used in *One Flew Over the Cuckoo's Nest*. This is now regarded with horror as disabling and brutal, but in the 1940s and 50s it was mainstream medicine. American doctors did about 40,000 of them as "cures" for schizophrenia, depression, and other mysterious disorders.

Is there anything bioethically amiss with mutilation, or deliberately inflicting a disability? At its most brutal there is the punishment of amputation – as in hands lopped off for theft under Sharia law. Less obviously disabling is chemical castration as a punishment for incorrigible sex offenders. We recoil from both of these because they make us just a bit less human.

However, a thief who has been maimed is still psychically normal. Chemical castration affects a paedophile's psyche by dulling his libido, but the procedure is reversible.

Things are different for the addict whose capacity for pleasure has been destroyed. He has been permanently mutilated both psychically and physically. He would be unable to appreciate a sunset, Mozart (or Lady Gaga), fine dining, the thrill of winning, the satisfaction of a job well done, the joy of hugging his children, his capacity for sexual intimacy. He would be just a husk of humanity, unrecognisable to his family and friends.

"To lesion this region that is thought to be involved in all types of motivation and pleasure risks crippling a human being," says Dr Charles O'Brien, head of the Center for Studies of Addiction at the University of Pennsylvania. David Linden, of Johns Hopkins, calls the surgery "horribly misguided."

Ablation of the nucleus accumbens is medicine only in the sense that capital punishment is a therapy for boredom. It removes the pain by removing the prisoner. Doctors are supposed to restore addicts' capacity to enjoy flourishing lives as human beings. This means helping them to regain self-mastery and set wholesome, realistic goals for themselves. The Chinese solution risks turning the addict from a man into a mouse. In the Odyssey, the enchantress Circe turned the companions of Odysseus into grunting swine. For Homer, 2,700 years ago, it seemed the most wretched of fates. It still is.

Part 10

Remember the great stem cell debate?

Nothing did more to put bioethics on the front page than the bitter disputes about human embryonic stem cells which opened the 21st century. Scientists have known since the 60s that some cells have the ability to change into various kinds of cells. The cell with the most potential is obviously the zygote – a single cell which eventually develops into every cell type in the body, from brain cells to fingernails to blood. In that cell are hidden the secrets of what the human body is and can be. Unlock them, and you may be able to abolish ageing, cure diseases and engineer the human genome. "The Promethean prospect of eternal regeneration awaits us, while time's vulture looks on," wrote one scientist at the height of the debate.

There is no doubt that a thorough understanding of stem cells could lead to amazing medical breakthroughs. But the problem was that human embryos had to be destroyed to create the cells with the most potential. Those who believe that a human being's life begins at fertilisation objected strongly. Those who didn't highlighted the incredible value of the research. The stage was set for huge debates in legislatures around the world.

Taken by our leaders

The Australian, 9 April 2002

What would Dr Spock say about the embryo debate?

Last week's embryo-politics show brought back memories of a great philosophical textbook, Star Trek. "Emotions are alien to me. I'm a scientist," Mr Spock would say without a flicker of a smile. And Captain Kirk would shake his head at the incapacity of his Vulcan sidekick to comprehend the simple experience of being human. Even in deep space there were debates about personhood.

Autistics such as Spock find it hard to distinguish people from things - rather like the Prime Minister and premiers at last week's Council of Australian Governments meeting, which authorised the use of surplus in-vitro fertilisation embryos for research. All John Howard needed was pointy Vulcan ears when he said: "I can't for the life of me see a moral difference between that [thawing the embryos] and the use of embryos in research."

The embryo debate proves that personhood is fragile. During the past 100 years, Jews, gypsies, blacks, homosexuals, counter-revolutionaries and Albanians have all been regarded as non-people unworthy of human rights. If these horrors have taught us anything, it is this: When personhood comes in many shades of grey, someone is going to get shafted.

For ethical autistics, humans are puzzling. Some are people; some are potential people; some used to be people. Vulcans have to carry around checklists of humanity-defining features such as size, self-consciousness, independence, and recognisable human shape. Embryos don't make the grade. This breaks with Australia's democratic traditions. We have always stood squarely with the humanism of *Star Trek*. In the words of "Bones" McCoy, the starship's doctor: "A *thing*? Why is something we don't understand always called a *thing*?"

Humans are what they are because of an unchanging nature that underlies changing appearances. You can no more have partial humanity than a partial triangle. There is no such thing as a pre-person stage of human life. Personhood begins at conception and lasts until death.

This is why the COAG meeting was so significant. For the first time, we have endorsed a Vulcan view of human nature as a checklist instead of an unchanging, constant, unified whole. This revolution has drawbacks that must be highlighted when the embryo bill goes before parliament.

The most obvious is that humanity and human rights have become negotiable. The embryo does not have enough ticks, so it will not be regarded as a person. In Spock's famous words: "It's life, Captain, but not life as we know it."

What about other humans without enough ticks, such as deformed babies or comatose patients? Vulcan philosopher Peter Singer has clear and simple ideas of what can be done. Is Howard prepared to tag along? And who ticks the boxes? Who will set the criteria for personhood or for what constitutes a worthwhile life?

So human life is now a source of profit. NSW Premier Bob Carr has compared IVF scientists with Galileo, but there is a difference: Galileo didn't have stock options.

If you want to peer into our future as a fully fledged Vulcan colony, look at China. Even ethically autistic politicians might have misgivings if they knew what is happening there.

Executions are the main source of organ transplants in China according to the *New York Times*. Last year, the 10,000 people put to death were put to good use - without their consent. Kidneys, livers, lungs, corneas and other organs were stripped from the prisoners and transplanted into wealthy patients. Like research on surplus embryos, this is a thrifty use of material that would otherwise be discarded.

China permits research on four-week-old embryos. The *Wall Street Journal* recently reported that Chinese scientists have cloned human embryos. Others have used rabbit egg cells to create them. "Eventually the fusion could lead to the development of a hybrid animal," said one of the scientists.

Could Australian ethical standards slip this low? Quite possibly. Earlier this month the vice-president of the Australian Medical Association, Trevor Mudge, defended stem cell research by asserting that "respect for human life is not an absolute". If Vulcan doctors abjure their Hippocratic oath, who can tell where we will end up?

Australians will be safer if they stick to the absolute value of human life at all stages of its cycle. To quote Kirk (Stardate 5431.6): "No one may kill a man. Not for any purpose. It cannot be condoned."

A Nobel Prize for stem cell ethics?

MercatorNet, 9 October 2012

This year's Nobel Prize for Medicine was shared by a Briton and a Japanese who respects the dignity of the human embryo.

Two stem cell researchers have shared the Nobel Prize in Medicine for 2012, an elderly Briton, Sir John B. Gurdon, and a younger Japanese, Shinya Yamanaka. By a serendipitous coincidence, Sir John made his discovery in 1962 – the year of Yamanaka's birth.

Fifty years of stem cell research have brought cures for intractable diseases within reach but they have also generated firestorms of controversy. Between 2001 and 2008, stem cell research vied with climate change as the most contentious issue in science. But since then, the firestorm died down -- basically because of Yamanaka's achievements. In fact, Tom Douglas, of the Uehiro Centre for Practical Ethics, at Oxford University, describes Yamanaka's work as "a rare example of a scientific discovery that may solve more ethical problems than it creates".

So what happened in these 50 years?

In his classic experiment at the University of Cambridge, Sir John discovered that cell development is reversible. The conventional wisdom was that cells could never change once they had specialized as nerve, skin, or muscle cells. He proved that this was wrong by replacing the nucleus of a frog egg cell with a nucleus from a mature intestinal cell. This modified cell developed into a normal tadpole.

This astonishing development eventually led to the cloning of the first mammal, Dolly the sheep, in 1996 and subsequent attempts by rogue scientists to clone human beings.

But while the technique clearly worked, no one really understood how cell development worked. The obvious target for research was the embryo. From this ball of undifferentiated cells come each of the body's specialized cells -- more than 200 of them in humans. Surely the answer must lie there. In 1998 an American scientist, James Thomson, of the University of Wisconsin-Madison, isolated and cultivated human embryonic stem cells.

But a one-eyed focus on embryos left stem cell science hostage to ethics. Despite scientists' bravado, everyone had some qualms about destroying embryos for their stem cells. Even Thomson admitted to the *New York Times* that "if human embryonic stem cell research does not make you at least a little bit uncomfortable, you have not thought about it enough".

Still, it seemed the only way forward. Desperate patient advocates, backed by a supporting chorus of bioethicists, scientists and doctors, argued tearfully that the possibility of miracle cures had to trump ethics.

But, in 2006, there came astonishing news from the University of Kyoto. An orthopaedic surgeon turned stem cell scientist, Shinya Yamanaka, had discovered that skin cells from mature mice could be reprogrammed to become immature stem cells. It was an amazingly imaginative step. Instead of mimicking natural development from embryo to adult, why not wind back the clock from adult to embryo?

Yamanaka found that by introducing only a few genes, specialized skin cells could become pluripotent stem cells, i.e. immature cells that can develop into all types of cells in the body. Until then, creating pluripotent cells without resorting to cloning seemed unlikely. Like Gurdon, for whom he has an immense respect, Yamanaka had skittled the conventional wisdom.

This was electrifying news for biologists. It was as if commuters on the pot-holed, terrorist-infested road from Baghdad airport to the Green Zone could suddenly detour down a six-lane autobahn at 200km. Many famous scientists dropped human embryonic stem cells and began work on what Yamanaka had termed "induced pluripotent stem cells". A year later, in November 2007, both he and James Thomson, in separate papers, confirmed that human cells could also be reprogrammed.

The rest is history.

As the Nobel Committee says about Gurdon and Yamanaka's research, "Textbooks have been rewritten and new research fields have been established. By reprogramming human cells, scientists have created new opportunities to study diseases and develop methods for diagnosis and therapy."

What turned Yamanaka away from the group-think which goaded his colleagues into the swamp of human embryonic stem cell research? Nowadays, the feverish excitement over human embryonic stem cells in the early Noughties seems ridiculous. Leading scientific and medical journals launched a crusade of Enlightenment heroes against prejudiced troglodytes. In one memorable endorsement of embryo research, the *New England Journal of Medicine* -- perhaps the world's leading medical journal -- published an editorial which concluded with this cringeworthy hyperbole: "The Promethean prospect of eternal regeneration awaits us, while time's vulture looks on." It never mentioned cell reprogramming.

Yamanaka's originality may have sprung from his ethical sensitivities. Even Julian Savulescu, the director of the Oxford

Uehiro Centre for Practical Ethics, who has no objections to embryo research, recognises this. "Yamanaka has taken people's ethical concerns seriously about embryo research and modified the trajectory of research into a path that is acceptable for all. He deserves not only a Nobel Prize for Medicine, but a Nobel Prize for Ethics."

In an interview with the New York Times in 2007, Yamanaka remembered one day years before when he paid a social visit to a friend's IVF clinic. There, he peered through a microscope. "When I saw the embryo, I suddenly realised there was such a small difference between it and my daughters," said the father of two. "I thought, we can't keep destroying embryos for our research. There must be another way."

Nor does he believe that scientists should put progress above ethics. In another 2007 interview, with *New Scientist*, he spoke about the firestorms. "These are very difficult decisions, and I think that society should make them," he said. "It should not be scientists. They can find it difficult to think like the person on the street, and instead may see it simply as a good opportunity. We scientists can be involved in the decision-making process, but I think unless society is comfortable with the therapy it should not go ahead."

Once again, experience shows that that ethical science is good science.

Back to taws on ethics

The Australian, 13 January 2006

The poster-boy of stem cell research is an out-and-out fraud

Stem cell scientists have been shattered by this week's confirmation that their poster boy, South Korean Hwang Woo-suk, is a fraud. Not Hwang alone, either. Many of his 24 co-authors on a landmark paper claiming to have cloned human embryos and created stem cell lines must have been accomplices. Storm clouds are gathering over Gerald Schatten, of the University of Pittsburgh, Hwang's co-author. The Korean president's chief science adviser, also a co-author, has resigned. Hwang may face criminal charges. It is one of the worst cases of scientific fraud in living memory.

Koreans wept. Scientists groaned. Patients felt betrayed. "I had pinned all my hopes on Dr Hwang after I heard that he had cured a dog with a spinal cord injury through stem cell treatment," paraplegic Park Seung-yoo told the *Joong Ahn Daily*. "I think about how I'm never going to walk again and I just want to die."

But in Australia, dreams blighted, money wasted, reputations shattered and research tainted are just a spot of bother. It's business as usual. "It's sad, but the field will move on," says the chief executive of the Australian Stem Cell Centre, Hugh Niall. "If anything, it's going to stimulate more research." And his colleague Martin Pera, agrees: "I don't think it will interfere with the progress of this work."

Hang on, guys. When the Columbia space shuttle disintegrated in 2003, NASA didn't sweep up the mess and book the next flight. It launched a two-year investigation before it tried again. And that's more or less what Australia should do with plans to legalise therapeutic cloning: shelve them.

What happened in Korea puts into question far more than the technology of therapeutic cloning. This has been delayed, but no doubt someone will eventually develop cloned stem cell lines. What Hwang's fraud has exposed is glaring systemic weaknesses involving this ethically controversial research, in which human embryos are created and destroyed for their stem cells.

First of all, its claims are consistently inflated by its practitioners. The first to clone an embryo, the American company Advanced Cell Technology, organised a media circus in 2001, which disgusted other scientists. A British group at the University of Newcastle was denounced by the journal *Nature* last year for rushing into print without peer review. Hwang is not the only stem cell scientist who wants to be a rock star. It's time for a bit of professional humility.

Second, journals such as *Science, The New England Journal of Medicine* and *Scientific American* are nakedly biased in favour of therapeutic cloning. That helps to explain why Hwang's faked results were not scrutinised carefully enough. "It is common knowledge that the bar for publication in this field often has appeared remarkably low, with even well-respected research journals seeming to fall over one another for the privilege of publishing the next hot paper," commented David Shaywitz, of the Harvard Stem Cell Institute, this week. It's time for some scientific objectivity.

Third, it is dismaying how easily governments are seduced by Amazing New Biotechnology Projects. Hwang didn't have to spike the drinks of Korean politicians to get them to pour millions into his research. They issued a postage stamp in his honour and anointed him "supreme scientist". Elsewhere it is no different. From Australia to Singapore to Britain to California, penny-pinching pollies who slash welfare budgets turn into sugar-daddy spendthrifts when they hear the words "embryonic stem cells". It's time to pour a bucket of cold water over our besotted politicians.

Fourth, and saddest, the public simply does not understand what is at stake, either ethically or scientifically. After the exposure of Hwang's lies about sourcing women's eggs for his experiments, hundreds of young women volunteered to donate their own, oblivious to the risks. Even this week, at the nadir of Hwang's reputation, hundreds of demonstrating fans displayed "Biotechnology Is Our Future" banners. Sixty-nine per cent of Koreans actually think that this manipulative liar and charlatan should be given a second chance. Is the Australian public really better informed? It's time for an intelligent public debate.

Finally, the Hwang affair suggests that when it comes to ethics, Australian stem cell scientists are not the sharpest knives in the drawer. For years they have said, and the media has repeated, that human embryos are no more than blobs of jelly. The public believed this because they were high-minded and successful. But now their celebrity colleagues have been exposed as shameless frauds moved by vanity, peer pressure, complacency and greed, just like the rest of us. Their embryo technology is still bogged at the starting line while adult stem cells have done several laps. What credibility can the crass utilitarianism that underlies this research have now? It's time to go back to taws on stem cell ethics.

Last month the Lockhart Review recommended that parliament legalise therapeutic cloning. In the light of what has happened in Korea, this would be a terrible blunder. It can no longer be business as usual for Australian stem cell research.

Not with a bang but a whimper
What ever happened to the stem cell wars?
MercatorNet, 3 November 2015

It's time for scientists and bioethicists to establish an Embryonic Stem Cell Truth and Reconciliation Commission.

It all seems so long ago now. But from 2002 to 2008 they barnstormed, fibbed, exaggerated, hyped, and caricatured to get government funding so that they could play God with human embryos. It was a brutal battle in which truth came second. "People need a fairy tale," said Ronald D.G. McKay, a leading stem cell scientist, in 2004.

The claims made for the near-miraculous potential of human embryonic stem cells were extraordinary. Celebrities and scientists spoke with the breathless enthusiasm normally associated with crystal medicine or ayurvedic medicine. Here are some, harvested at random:

> If we cannot become Titans using our own stem-cell resources, perhaps we can resist the onslaught of time's vulture by transplanting pluripotent cells derived from early embryos to supplement our own waning supplies of stem cells. --*Nadia Rosenthal, in the New England Journal of Medicine, 2003.*

> "Science has presented us with a hope called stem-cell research, which may provide our scientists with answers that have so long been beyond our grasp. I just don't see how we can turn our backs on this, there are just so many diseases that can be cured, or at least helped. We have lost so much time already, and I just really can't bear to lose any more." – *Former First Lady Nancy Reagan*

> "Personally, I can't think of a greater affirmation of the culture

of life than to advance the fight against disease by increasing federal funding for biomedical research. Equally crucial is to remove undue restrictions on important paths forward, including embryonic stem cell research. America is about optimism, about promise, about always moving forward. The idea of rejecting one of the most promising areas of research is short-sighted."
– *Michael J. Fox, Founder, Michael J. Fox Foundation for Parkinson's Research*

"It is difficult to estimate just how damaging the current restrictions have been to the field to date, but if the current restrictions are not eventually lifted, patients will suffer needlessly." – *James Thomson of the University of Wisconsin, Madison*

"The U.S. House of Representatives has voted to ban research on, and the use of, medical treatments derived from embryonic stem cells. This bill is short-sighted and has the potential to put many critical future advances in medicine beyond the reach of patients in the United States." – *Jeffrey Drazen, Editor, New England Journal of Medicine*

Foes of embryo research were called troglodytes and religious fundamentalists; they were frauds waging war on genuine science. Their scientific credentials were questioned. They were accused of being callous and indifferent to the suffering of patients with chronic illness.

And yet they were right. Not one person has been cured with embryonic stem cells. Not one.

The controversy ran out of steam almost immediately after Japanese researcher Shinya Yamanaka developed induced pluripotent stem cells (iPS cells) in 2007, a feat for which he was later awarded the Nobel Prize in Medicine. His cells apparently have all the potential of embryonic cells without the ethical baggage. Leading scientists quietly stopped working with hES cells and moved to the new cells.

Nonetheless, some scientists still insisted that hES cells were the gold standard; destructive embryo research would always be essential for the advancement of science.

Now, in the concluding act of the stem cell wars, a paper in *Biotechnology* has suggested that iPS cells and hES cells are functionally equivalent – effectively meaning that there is no need to destroy embryos either for research or for therapies. If it is true – and it needs to be confirmed by other researchers – it is the stem cell equivalent of receiving the surrender of the last Japanese soldier on some remote island in the Philippines. Whether or not the findings of Konrad Hochedlinger and colleagues at Massachusetts General Hospital in Boston are correct, the war is over.

However, a news report in *Science* of this finding has attracted not one single comment. This attitude is thoroughly dishonourable. All those eminent journal editors, journalists, scientists, bioethicists, and politicians who insisted that destructive embryo research was vital were wrong. Will there be no apology?

11

Reporting bioethics news

Most people receive both their moral guidance and their facts through the media. Hence journalists ought to realise that they have a special responsibility for ensuring that their articles are well researched and frame ethical debates in an intelligent way. Sadly, this is often not the case. Journalists may simply not have the scientific or philosophical background to understand and explain complex scenarios. But there are other problems as well. They may be intimidated by scientific flim-flam; they may be tone-deaf ethically; they may even be foot-soldiers in a crusade to change ethical standards. Whatever the problem, I believe that we all need to be more sceptical of men and women in white coats preaching about their visions of a brighter future for humanity.

The Economist's moral blinkers

MercatorNet, 25 November 2006

Many people have traded in their brains for a subscription to world's best news magazine. Are they better off?

Plus ça change, plus c'est la même chose. A few months ago, Bill Emmott, the editor of *The Economist*, retired after 13 years at the helm of the world's best news magazine. He was replaced by the US editor, John Micklethwait. There was a flurry of reports in the media and then their names disappeared under the blanketing snow of current affairs. As part of the 163-year-old tradition, no by-lines appear in *The Economist*, not even the name of its editor. The next time Mr Micklethwait's name will appear could be his own retirement.

More than a magazine, *The Economist* is an institution – a relic of the Victorian era founded upon the economics of Adam Smith and the morals of John Stuart Mill which has adapted superbly to modern times. In the post-modern age of fragmentation and doubt its business is certitude. But with flair: its covers are often hilarious; its style sober, garnished with sly humour. Headlines in Latin pop up from time to time; allusions to Shakespeare and English poets pepper the text. It is supremely readable and entertaining. Originally British, during Mr Emmott's watch, *The Economist* prospered across the Atlantic and turned a good reputation into an outstanding brand. Half of its circulation of one million is now in the United States. Mr Micklethwait will no doubt ensure the continuity of its free market philosophy and maintain its high standards of editing.

"I used to think. Now, I just read *The Economist*," Larry Ellison,

CEO of IT giant Oracle Corporation, has admitted. The list of political and business luminaries who read it religiously is long and impressive. "The magazine I spend most of my days reading is *The Economist*," says Microsoft's Bill Gates. "An important part of my life support system," says Chris Patten, Chancellor of Oxford University.

Even its rivals are glowing in their praise. Here's the *International Herald Tribune*: "This unique journal in which sheer intellect, backed by integrity and a bold welcoming of new ideas has held sway over statesman and governments." And Germany's *Die Zeit*: "The paper of the global ruling classes." And if you're still not convinced, Vanity Fair: "The magazine is probably read by more presidents, prime ministers, and chief executives around the world than any other... The positions it takes change the minds that matter."

Which makes it all the more disturbing when *The Economist* takes up the cudgels in favour of infant euthanasia. The UK's Royal College of Obstetricians and Gynaecologists has suggested that the rights and wrongs of actively killing disabled infants should be debated. It is hardly surprising that doctors paid to kill infants on one side of the birth canal should seek permission to kill them on the other side, too. But it seems odd that the world's most respected magazine should swallow their arguments and drizzle them with treacly sentimentality: "Tiny babies do tug at the heartstrings but raising a severely impaired child is heartbreakingly hard. It is brave of doctors to dare to question whether they should save the life of each and every one."

Brave? How about immoral? How about cowardly? How about inhuman? How could the world's best news magazine be so wrong-headed about killing babies?

The Economist prides itself upon "its objective, factual writing, rather than... emotive journalism", but on nearly every important moral issue, the ghost of John Stuart Mill whispers that morality must be dismissed as an inconvenient superstition. Should the West shower Africa with condoms to prevent AIDS? Naturally -- "morality must take second place". Same sex marriage? Obviously -- "The case for allowing gays to marry begins with equality, pure and simple." Legalise prostitution? Why not? "What consenting adults do in private is their own business." Should Olympians take drugs? -- It is "shrill" and "intolerant" to suggest otherwise. And so on.

Despite the vast common sense and analytical clarity of its business and political analysis, *The Economist* wears the ideological blinkers of a Victorian free-thinker. It racks moral arguments on the Procrustean bed of Mill's libertarianism. For instance, the author of one of its excellent surveys defends the legalisation of illegal drugs by citing the great man: "The only purpose for which power can be rightfully exercised over any member of a civilised community, against his will, is to prevent harm to others." Like Mill, *The Economist* regards the person as an autonomous, self-sufficient individual who shapes his own good without reference to society. Furthermore, for *The Economist*, the market is not a way to achieve the good of society; it is the good of society. Any social policy which introduces a market or makes a market more efficient is to be praised. Any one which does not is to be censured as antiquated and moralistic.

It is hard to find a better example of how ideology colours the magazine's vaunted objectivity than its recent leader (*The Economist* has "leaders", not editorials) defending a market in which people could sell their kidneys for profit. It would be safer for patients and it would eliminate long waiting lists. "Instinct often trumps logic. Sometimes that's right. But in this case, the instinct that selling bits of oneself is wrong leads to many premature deaths and much suffering. The logical answer, in this case, is the humane one."

But this is ideological, rather than logical. How does *The Economist* justify itself? By using as a case study a place where the sale of kidneys has been legalised, where donors are amply compensated and where waiting lists have been eliminated: Iran. It's perplexing to see a country with one of the world's worst records on human rights used to justify a policy which puts human rights at risk.

And the argument is not confined to the leader, but seeps into the news coverage as well. The contrary view -- that donors' health is compromised, that they will be exploited, that it will not stop the black market -- is ignored. Even though it admits that "there is little information on how donors ultimately fare," *The Economist* still accepts the glib assurances of the Iranian brokers that donors remain healthy. But isn't the ultimate health of the donors the central issue in the debate over selling kidneys? As often happens, *The Economist's* evidence often looks threadbare and its arguments unravel when they are teased apart.

The plausibility of a market for organs and other such proposals owes more to a team of brilliant editors than to logic and evidence. *The Economist's* reputation for omniscience and its tightly-written, sardonic style anaesthetise criticism. While by-lines in other magazines and newspapers reveal the name of journalists and allow readers to imagine that bias and misinformation -- not to mention disinformation -- might be possible, its Olympian anonymity reinforces the myth that it has canvassed all points of view, sifted all the evidence and formed a dispassionate opinion.

This is nonsense, of course. All journalism reflects the ethical prejudices of an author – even at *The Economist*. Back in the late 50s, readers were probably not aware that its Middle East correspondent was Kim Philby, a spy who did incalculable damage to Britain and the United States and was eventually buried in Moscow with the honours of a KGB general. Had they known, perhaps they might have treated *The Economist's* pronouncements on the Middle East with just a bit more scepticism. As The Economist itself might put it, if you are thinking of trading in your brain for a subscription, *caveat emptor*.

Kowtowing to Planned Parenthood

MercatorNet, 3 August 2015

What has happened to the crusading zeal of the New York Times?

A team of a team of undercover freelance investigative journalists called the Center for Medical Progress has been making life miserable for abortion provider Planned Parenthood over the past few weeks.

It has released four videos in which senior figures in Planned Parenthood calmly discuss the market in foetal parts for scientific research. There are stomach-churning scenes of laboratory workers carefully sifting through shreds of a tiny human body for commercially valuable material.

As advocacy, videos are brilliant. "I think [the first video is] totally an A+," communications expert Yoel Inbar, of the University of Toronto, told *New York Magazine*. "The way that the Planned Parenthood doctor talks about this, it doesn't do them any favours. I'm pro-choice personally, but I thought it was a little creepy."

Planned Parenthood has vehemently denied that it is breaking any laws by supplying human hearts, livers, brains and other organs. But after watching the videos some Senators and Congressmen are vowing to do everything they can to defund the organisation, even if it means shutting down the government. (Admittedly, they are all Republicans.) At stake is more than US$500 million in Planned Parenthood's funding from the government.

David Daleiden, the spokesman for the CMP, says that several more videos are on the way, although courts have slapped two injunctions on the group to keep it from releasing them.

This kind of power and publicity is every journalist's dream. When Julian Assange and Edward Snowden illegally released confidential government documents, they appeared on the front page of *Time* magazine. The editorialised about Snowden's leaks: "He may have committed a crime to do so, but he has done his country a great service." It argued that he should be pardoned or just given a slap on the wrist so that he could continue to speak truth to power.

For the record, I didn't support the actions of Assange or Snowden and don't support Daleiden's deceptive tactics either. In the long run, breaking the law (or stretching it to the breaking point) is going to be counterproductive. Still, the information gathered by all three has exposed shocking abuses. And in the case of the CMP videos, even fervent supporters of "legal, safe and rare" abortion will be revolted by the commodification of human life.

How did the *Times* respond?

Very strangely. In the strongest possible language, it denounced Daleiden and his comrades as the Voldemorts of "women's reproductive rights" and worst of all, of being, um, journalists. "The Center for Medical Progress video campaign is a dishonest attempt to make legal, voluntary and potentially lifesaving tissue donations appear nefarious and illegal."

Well, actually, that's not quite the case. It's an attempt to see whether the donations are *in fact* legal and voluntary. Journalists tend to do that sort of thing. Being sceptical about bland reassurances from organisations with budgets of over $1 billion is widely recognised as part of their job description.

This clothes peg-on-the-nose attitude is odd for a newspaper whose motto is "All the News That's Fit to Print". And even odder for a newspaper which thumbed its nose at the might of the US government over whistleblowers like Daniel Ellsberg, Julian Assange, and Edward Snowden. In its most recent justification of illegal revelations it argued that:

> Mr. Snowden was clearly justified in believing that the only way to blow the whistle on this kind of intelligence-gathering was to expose it to the public and let the resulting furore do the work his superiors would not.

Large organisations like the National Security Agency (or Planned Parenthood) tend to deny that they ever have done, are doing or ever will do anything which is nefarious and illegal. That's what their public relations staff are paid to say. Real journalists, on the other hand, are paid not to take what they say at face value.

Even if the *Times* supports abortion, it should still probe Planned Parenthood's good intentions. The United States had the best of intentions when it invaded Iraq. And then there was Abu Ghraib... It is tragic that America's paper of record has become an unpaid extension of Planned Parenthood's PR office.

The Lancet stumbles over assisted dying

MercatorNet, 7 September 2015

Editor's attack based on anti-Christian prejudice

At long last, Richard Horton, editor-in-chief of *The Lancet*, appears to have made up his mind about "assisted dying" in the United Kingdom, a few days before Parliament votes on a private member's bill this week.

As he pointed out in the Comment section of his journal, "Careful readers of *The Lancet* may have noticed that we have had little to say about assisted dying (or physician-assisted suicide) in recent years. Moral cowardice? Perhaps more that we couldn't easily make our minds up."

Dr Horton's article is not a ringing endorsement of the bill. But in his carefully worded assessment of its safeguards he rings no alarm bells and he underscores his perception that there is a "growing consensus" on the issue.

Altogether, it is a world away from his position in 2006. Back then, commenting on another assisted dying bill, he wrote: "A commitment to life may present troubling dilemmas to the modern physician; but a commitment to death will undermine the very nature of doctoring itself."

Editors are free to change their minds without explaining why. Unhappily, this is not a courtesy that Dr Horton has extended to Baroness Ilora Finlay, whom he describes as "the most high-profile campaigner against assisted dying" in the UK. Baroness Finlay is the immediate past president of the British Medical Association and a leading palliative care physician. She obviously knows more than most of us about death and dying. Possibly more than the editor of *The Lancet*.

Yet Dr Horton slyly suggests that the real reason why she opposes assisted dying is her religious beliefs. "Some of those resisting changes to the law do so by deliberately using speculative and misleading arguments—'fibbing for God'," he writes.

Funny about that. In her eloquent essay against assisted dying in *The Economist* earlier this year, Baroness Finlay put forward powerful arguments. I have no idea what her religious beliefs are, but they weren't needed to make her case.

If the sharpest arrow in Dr Horton's quiver is to insinuate that his opponents are insincere and tainted by a faith which he does not share, his others must be blunt indeed. Personally, I can't understand this prurient interest in people's religious lives. Arguments stand or fall on their merits, not on conjectural links to extramural activities. One might as well attribute Sartre's atheism to his chain-smoking or Berkeley's idealism to his chronic constipation. But if you handed these famous philosophers nicotine patches and laxatives, I doubt whether they would alter their arguments.

The idea that religious convictions invalidate arguments based on evidence and reason has several problems.

One, it is a slur on the character of people like Baroness Finlay. To assert that she is deliberately advancing an argument in which she does not believe in order to enforce a policy with which she does agree means that she is thoroughly dishonest. Could a creature of such low morals really become president of the BMA? A canard like this is simply not credible.

Second, it is a slur on her readers who, it is assumed, are too stupid to recognise the bait-and-switch.

Third, there is no such thing as a policy without a cultural foundation, whether it be Christianity or atheism. Christians believe in the supreme value of life. Atheists believe in the meaninglessness of life. Both philosophies influence a discussion of assisted dying.

Fourth, in any case, the mantra of the assisted dying movement, "my life, my death, my choice", is not based on evidence and reason. It is chanted by ideologues whose faith in radical autonomy is more religious than rational. We did not bring ourselves into life; we have not maintained ourselves in life; and whether we may choose death regardless of the common good is debatable.

Fifth, the idea that Christians should retire from public life precisely because they are Christians is absurd. If everyone with convictions were to be disenfranchised, the British electorate would shrink to almost nothing. Only three categories of voters would remain: the brain-dead, the psychopaths, and video-gamers role-playing the first two.

Dismissing arguments because their authors are religious is basically a grown-up version of playground name-calling. The debate over assisted dying is too serious for that. Let's stick to reason and evidence.

Tabloid bioethics

Australasian Science, September 2011

Tabloid journalism gives bioethical issues the social relevance that academic debates lack.

By the time you read this, the volcanic ash from the eruption of public outrage over phone-hacking in Rupert Murdoch's tabloids may have dissipated. I am writing this the day after he appeared before a committee of the British Parliament and acknowledged that it was "the most humble day of my life". The ethics of his tabloid newspapers may have mortally wounded his company.

Factoids, trendoids, paranoids and haemorrhoids: tabloids keep good company in the dictionary. There has never been any secret about the degrading moral qualities of the *News of the World* and competitors like *The Sun*, the *Daily Mail* and the *Daily Express*. They were bottom-feeders sucking up everything that was tasteless, prurient, salacious and vulgar in British life. Their lifeblood was the invasion of celebrities' privacy.

But, as a reporter of things bioethical, I'd like to put in a good word for the tabloids on their day of shame, or SHAME!!!! as they might put it. At this juncture, I feel compelled to insert a disclaimer: neither I nor any family member hold, nor have I or any family members ever held, shares in any company related to News Corp. With that over, let me attempt to rinse a bit of the dirt from the besmirched reputation of yellow journalism.

All ethical disciplines, especially bioethics, are about how people should act. They involve a great deal of theorising in academic journals like *Bioethics*, the *Journal of Medical Ethics* and *the*

Hastings Center Report. There are vigorously competing theories – principalism, utilitarianism, virtue ethics, natural law ethics, Kantian deontology and so on.

No matter which corner of the ring the professional bioethicist is in, someone else is in the other corner, gloves up, spoiling for a fight to the death over the legitimacy of preference utilitarianism. But the rush of blood in an academic bunfight all too often bleaches out the real-life people behind bioethical debates – the deathbed gasps of your grandmother, a neighbour's lingering battle with cancer, the childlessness of the woman in the next bed. And the London tabloids have no peer in conveying the human consequences of dry bioethics debates.

Bioethicists do pencil sketches that highlight features relevant to their particular theory. But the best tabloid reporters paint in oils, adding as much colour and lurid detail as possible.

Some are better than others, of course. I cannot recall (there's a familiar line!) ever sourcing a story for my bioethics newsletter from the *News of the World*. But the *Daily Mail*, which has positioned itself as a "middle-market" tabloid, consistently does an excellent job of giving a three-dimensional picture of ethical conundrums.

Let me give an example. Last year a headline in the *Daily Mail* announced: "I'm trying for Bin Laden's grandchild: Briton's surrogacy deal with son of terror chief". After reading this story, anyone with a bit of grey matter must wonder whether the desire for a child is enough to justify surrogacy.

Three people were involved. Twenty-nine-year-old Omar bin Laden, fourth son of Osama, is as rich as Croesus. But for some reason he ended up as the sixth husband of 54-year-old Jane Felix-Browne, now known as Zaina Mohamad al-Sabah bin

Laden after her conversion to Islam. She is a grandmother who suffers from multiple sclerosis and has three adult children from her previous relationships.

Zaina's biological clock rang midnight long ago, but the couple wanted a baby. So they engaged 24-year-old Louise Pollard, a former pole-dancer whose ambition is to become Britain's most prolific surrogate.

The *Daily Mail* reported that Ms Pollard had time for recreation at a secret bolt-hole in the Middle East. "At one point I was sitting there playing Call of Duty on the PlayStation with Omar and I just sat there and thought, I'm playing video games with Osama Bin Laden's son! How random is that?"

It's fashionable to be non-judgemental (except about the absolute evil of phone-hacking) but surely the stability and maturity of these three amigos deserves to be "interrogated", to use a word from bioethics jargon. The tabloids do, implicitly; the journals don't.

A good tabloid reporter gets people to talk and talk and talk. This spew of consciousness is not judged or theorised. It's served up juicy and raw.

But sometimes, perhaps not too often but certainly sometimes, tabloids make you think.

The tangled knot of the last taboo
MercatorNet, 12 April 2016

Now that incest has been rebadged as 'genetic sexual attraction', will it be legalised?

The British press is a fathomless mine of lurid but thought-provoking, strange-but-true explorations of the dark side of the human condition. Last week's revelation was published in a magazine called *The New Day* -- a passionate incestuous romance between a 51-year-old British woman and her 32-year-old American son.

Kim West was studying in California when she had a child out of wedlock. She gave him up for adoption and turned to England. Nearly 30 years later she learned that her son Ben Ford wanted to contact her. When they met, they immediately felt an overwhelming sexual attraction. Ben ended up abandoning his wife and moving in with his mother. They live together and are considering having children.

Post-adoption romance is a poorly-understood but well-documented phenomenon. In 1980s an American adoption counsellor, Barbara Gonyo, coined the term "genetic sexual attraction"(GSA) for these passionate feelings. Two British psychologists interviewed several people in the grip of GSA who all described "a romantic 'falling in love', intense and explosive, sudden and almost irresistible".

Since incest is not only taboo but illegal in most jurisdictions, people are reluctant to discuss it. However, the psychologists estimated that such feeling are present about 50 percent of the time when siblings and parents are reunited. Their article was published 20 years ago in the *British Journal of Medical Psychology* (later renamed *Psychology and Psychotherapy*), so it is possible that the number of cases has increased.

In fact, as a sympathetic columnist for The (London) *Telegraph* pointed out, the use of anonymous sperm donation could cause a huge increase in the prevalence of GSA. Children can contact their biological parents as soon as they turn 18 in the UK, so numbers are bound to grow as "genetic orphans" seek out the parents they have never seen. She concluded that:

> Those who succumb to GSA are not sickos, or freaks, but victims who desperately need help and understanding. Their feelings are not controllable, but with scientific research and support, we can give them some degree in control over this devastating affliction.

Do these reasons for sympathising with GSA ring a bell? – there is an irresistible love; the "victims" are genetically hard-wired and helpless; it is increasingly common, and, possibly more socially acceptable.

Aren't these precisely the same reasons which have buttressed the legalisation of homosexuality and same-sex marriage? If the defining characteristic of love is erotic impulse, it is only logical to legalise incest as well.

Legal arguments are already being rolled out. In an article in the journal *Criminal Law and Philosophy*, an academic at Rutgers School of Law, Vera Bergelson, has argued that the traditional reasons for banning incest are over or under-inclusive, inconsistent or clearly inadequate. For instance, when pressed, opponents of incest argue that children are harmed. But she responds that science does not bear this out:

> ... it is far from clear that inbreeding presents a threat to

society. The number of serious genetic disorders associated with inbreeding is quite limited. Moreover, some scientists believe that, in the long run, populations may suffer from the prevention of consanguineous marriages ...

In any case, a higher probability of genetic defects is hardly a reason to ban marriage. If that were the case, society would ban IVF, which has an elevated rate of birth defects. She concludes, as supporters of homosexuality did in the 1970s:

> the true reason behind the long history of the incest laws is the feeling of repulsion and disgust this tabooed practice tends to evoke in the majority of population. However, in the absence of wrongdoing, neither a historic taboo nor the sense of repulsion and disgust legitimizes criminalization of an act.

Having accepted the logic of same-sex marriage, it is difficult to reject the logic of legalised incest. All we need is GSA's answer to Caitlyn/Bruce Jenner – a glamorous couple who are hopelessly in "love". Stay tuned for a campaign for GSA Rights.

Cracks in the edifice of science

Australasian Science, July/August 2012

A tenfold increase in the number of retractions over the past 10 years raises questions about the infallibility of peer review of scientific research.

The novels of Sinclair Lewis (1885–1951), the first American Nobel laureate for literature, seem rather clunky nowadays but he had a knack for channelling the *Zeitgeist*. In *Arrowsmith*, published in 1925, an old German professor eulogises scientists:

> The normal man, he does not care much what he does except that he should eat and sleep and make love. But the scientist is intensely religious – he is so religious that he will not accept quarter-truths, because they are an insult to his faith. He wants that everything should be subject to inexorable laws... He is the only real revolutionary.

Decades later, the public still regards men and women in white lab coats as selfless seekers after truth. However, some thoughtful scientists are worried. Even though the scientific method is universally accepted as one of mankind's greatest achievements, it has been bruised by the all-too-human failings: greed, aggression, fraud, and ambition.

In fact, some speak of a crisis.

The *New York Times* recently highlighted the belief of the editor of the scientific journal Infection and Immunity, Dr Ferric C. Fang, that a tenfold increase in the number of retractions over the past 10 years is a symptom of "a dysfunctional scientific climate".

Fang recently issued a call for root-and-branch reform in an eloquent editorial:

> Incentives in the current system place scientists under tremendous stress, discourage cooperation, encourage poor scientific practices, and deter new talent from entering the field. It is time for a discussion of how the scientific enterprise can be reformed to become more effective and robust.

He pointed to familiar problems: gender imbalance, the imperative of publish or perish, cheating and blatant fraud, selective reporting of results, the race to publish first, celebrity science and so on. "The present system," he wrote, "provides... potent incentives for behaviours that are detrimental to science and scientists".

In an opinion piece in *Nature*, the co-director of the Consortium for Science, Policy and Outcomes at Arizona State University, Dr Daniel Sarewitz, spoke of "alarming cracks" that are undermining public trust. "Science's internal controls on bias [are] failing, and bias and error [are] trending in the same direction – towards the pervasive over-selection and over-reporting of false positive results."

Significantly for bioethics, he said that "the cracks in the edifice are showing up first in the biomedical realm, because research results are constantly put to the practical test of improving human health".

Even the peer review process, commonly regarded as the gold standard for trustworthiness, is being questioned. In recent years spectacular research frauds have slipped through reviewers for the world's best journals. Hwang Woo Suk, a disgraced Korean stem cell expert whose work was published in *Nature* and *Science*, and Andrew Wakefield, an autism expert whose discredited research was published in *The Lancet*, spring to mind.

The UK government, which finances much of British research, actually held a Parliamentary inquiry into peer review last year. While it broadly endorsed the current system, the report brought to light some surprising dissenters.

Drummond Rennie, deputy editor of the *Journal of the American Medical Association*, once said: "If peer review was a drug it would never be allowed onto the market".

And Richard Horton, editor-in-chief of *The Lancet*, quoted approvingly a study which said: "Editorial peer review, although widely used, is largely untested and its effects are uncertain".

There are influential contemporary philosophers who believe that knowledge is so tainted by our own biases that it is impossible to attain truth and objectivity about anything, from music to astronomy. This is might just be post-modernist twaddle, but these small cracks in the edifice of science do suggest that more modesty about the authority of lab coats would be welcome in public debates.

Thundering "the science has spoken" – about the potential of embryonic stem cells, about the health of IVF children, about post-abortion trauma and a host of other bioethical issues – does not mean that all debate must come to an end.

A bizarre dilemma from Sweden

Australasian Science, April 2016

"Resignation syndrome" in refugee children and adolescents in Sweden is one of the strangest medical stories of the past decade

The political and policing problems of allowing hundreds of thousands of refugees from Africa, the Middle East, and Afghanistan to plod into Western Europe tend to overshadow the difficulties of settling them into a new and alien society.

On the medical front countries in Western Europe are well prepared to cope with the massive influx, according to the World Health Organization. But inevitably there are exotic health issues. Female genital mutilation is one that has made headlines. One that hasn't is "resignation syndrome" in refugee children and adolescents in Sweden.

This must be one of the most bizarre medical stories of the past decade, although it has received almost no publicity outside of Sweden. Hundreds of children and teenagers, aged 7 to 19, have been diagnosed with a mysterious ailment which leaves them unable to eat, speak and move. According to an article by Dr Karl Sallin and colleagues *in Frontiers of Behavioural Neuroscience*, the typical patient is "totally passive, immobile, lacks tonus, [is] withdrawn, mute, unable to eat and drink, incontinent and not reacting to physical stimuli or pain".

Unless they are given intensive nursing care, they will die.

And it happens only in Sweden.

In 2014 Swedish medical authorities started calling the

phenomenon "resignation syndrome", but this is just a label, not a solution. All of the affected children are members of ethnic minorities, many of them from former Soviet republics, with a disproportionate share being Uighurs. Many of them have been traumatised by experiencing domestic abuse, witnessing violence or being harassed. But only children from refugee families are affected; unaccompanied children are not.

None of the conventional explanations hold water. It could be a reaction to stress and trauma. It could be a projection of the anxieties of traumatised mothers. But there are 50 million traumatised refugees scattered all over the world. Why does "resignation syndrome" happen only in Sweden?

Dr Sallin proposes a two-fold diagnosis in his article. He argues that the affected children are actually suffering from an old and well-studied ailment: catatonia. They are conscious, but unable to move or respond, even to painful stimuli.

His second point is more controversial. He maintains that it is a kind of mass hysteria. Jean-Martin Charcot, a French neurologist in the late 19th century, was the first to characterise this phenomenon. The symptoms of his patients, mostly women, were recurring fits, often quite bizarre, which seemed to follow a standard path of growing severity.

After ruling out a physical cause, he concluded that the cause was psychological, and the ailment was transmitted by imitating other people's hysterics. When the symptoms became "unfashionable", the hysterical fits declined. Sallin believes that symptoms of hysteria evolve over time "through the continuous negotiation between physicians and patients immersed in cultural context".

This leads him to suggest that the refugee children are

suffering from a mass psychogenic illness tailored for people in their community, just as in past outbreaks:

> Highly segregated groups where stress, control or obligations are evident and inescapable are predisposed and historically in particular religious settings are overrepresented. Female patients predominate. Patients below 20 years of age are overrepresented. Epidemics involve typical symptoms, including fatigue and unconsciousness, without demonstrable organic lesions. Relapse is common. 'Compensational' issues have been reported of importance. Media reports are known to enable transmission of illness behaviour.

So this leads us to the bioethical angle to this strange phenomenon. Publicising the illness in the media may make the public more aware of a pressing public health issue, but it may be spreading it at the same time. And indeed it appears that there was a peak in cases of "resignation syndrome" when it was given extensive coverage in the media.

So Sallin concludes with a morose reflection upon the dilemma that doctors find themselves in. As physicians they are bound to tube-feed their catatonic patients, but caring for them may cause the syndrome to spread even further: "The appeal to culture-bound psychopathology raises an ethical dilemma … by offering treatment, to which there is no alternative, we are also, on another level, causing new cases."

Part 12

Peering into the future

There's a mantra repeated by journalists around the world whenever they report a scientific breakthrough: technology is racing ahead and ethics are lagging behind. There is a bit of truth in this. Take a development like driverless cars. They are so novel that there are bound to be many unanswered questions. Can machines be trusted? How should they be programmed to act if a smash is inevitable? Who is responsible for the damage: the driver or the manufacturer? And so on. The ethical analysis is lagging behind.

But it is wrong to say that the ethics are lagging behind. Before and after driverless cars, the lives of innocent human beings are still more important than the destruction of inanimate property. Fundamental principles do not change. We just need the practical wisdom to know how to apply them.

The end is nigh!
MercatorNet, 12 May 2016

Oxford researchers say that there is a 9.5% chance of the extinction of humanity in the next hundred years.

I have not been blessed with a refined taste in cinema, with my favourite movie franchise being the *Terminator* series, especially the second and third, in which Arnie is in peak form. Alas, there's not enough space here to reminisce, so let's confine ourselves to the premise for the action.

On August 29, 1997, Skynet, an artificial intelligence system created by the US Defense Department, became self-conscious. Its programmers panicked and tried to deactivate it. Skynet defended itself by provoking a nuclear exchange in which three billion people died and the rest were enslaved or hunted down. Until John Connor organised the Resist…

Sorry, we must stop here as I've promised to talk about ethics.

Surprisingly, a minor academic industry exists whose goal is to solve the conundrums which might arise if (or when) Skynet or one of its buddies takes over the world. And this is just one of many apocalyptic scenarios which are on the table. The Global Priorities Project and the Future of Humanity Institute, both based at Oxford University, recently produced a Global Catastrophic Risk 2016 report which discusses some of the most likely ones.

It's less gripping than the Left Behind novels about the Second Coming (with titles like *The Rapture: In the Twinkling of an Eye* or

Countdown to the Earth's Last Days), but, in its own dry, detached way, no less scary.

According to the Oxford experts' calculations, extinction of the whole human race is reasonably likely. Scientists have suggested that the risk is 0.1% per year, and perhaps as much as 0.2%. While this may not seem worthwhile worrying about, these figures actually imply, says the report, that "an individual would be more than five times as likely to die in an extinction event than a car crash".

Tiny probabilities add up, so that the chance of extinction in the next century is 9.5% -- which is worth worrying about. And of course, a mere global catastrophe, involving the death of a tenth of the population, is far more likely.

What sort of events do the futurists have in mind? The first of them has been on the front page of newspapers for several years: extreme climate change.

Then there is nuclear warfare, which would not only kill millions, but possibly trigger a nuclear winter. Pandemics like the Spanish Flu in 1918-19 have already killed millions. Natural events like the eruption of a supervolcano or a collision with an asteroid would be extremely challenging, as the dinosaurs discovered.

But what worries the futurists most is the risk of "emerging technologies" such as Skynet in The Terminator. Oxford's Nick Bostrom, a philosopher from Sweden, is the leading light in the study of existential risk. In his recent book Superintelligence: Paths, Dangers, Strategies, he contends that artificial intelligence could become as powerful as the human mind, with a small, but hardly negligible, risk of something like Skynet developing. (Its message comes "highly recommended" by Bill Gates, which suggests that the world's richest man is not secretly planning to take over the world with a Microsoft version of Skynet.)

There are other runaway technologies which could destroy us. A killer microbe could be created with genetic engineering techniques which could wipe out whole populations. Colossal attempts to alter the climate with geoengineering techniques could backfire and turn the planet into desert or a snowfield. And then there are all the dangers which we foolishly don't fear because we don't even realise that they exist.

What, for instance, is the probability of Vogons showing up to build a hyperspatial express route through our star system? In *A Hitchhiker's Guide to the Galaxy*, it took slightly less than two minutes to demolish planet earth and only two people survived.

So here's where futurology stops and ethics begins: what should society do about massively destructive events with a low probability?

This is a question which is relatively recent, philosophically speaking. People began to pose it in the 1960s because of the threat of "mutually assured destruction" in a nuclear exchange, the imagined dangers of over-population, and climate change.

Nick Bostrom advises us not to wait for the worst to happen. He believes that "a moral case can be made that existential risk reduction is strictly more important than any other global public good."

After doing a probability analysis of risk and future populations, he comes to the conclusion that "the expected value of reducing existential risk by a mere one billionth of one billionth of one percentage point is worth a hundred billion times as much as a billion human lives". This is difficult to comprehend, but the conclusion isn't: "the objective of reducing existential risks should be a dominant consideration whenever we act out of an impersonal concern for humankind as a whole".

In other words, we can never do enough to save humanity.

Personally, I find this blank cheque even scarier than supervolcanoes. It implies that governments should be empowered to tax to the max, spend freely, revise moral codes and restrict civil liberties to save humanity from invisible threats.

But is it sensible to entrust our future to statisticians? After all, calculations are only as good as the assumptions on which they are based. The old computing proverb, garbage in, garbage out, has yet to be disproved. It is easy to make enormous mistakes by moving a decimal point or neglecting to consider important inputs.

For instance, Paul Ehrlich confidently predicted that "hundreds of millions" would starve to death in the 1970s. This helped to create a world-wide panic over the "population bomb". To avert catastrophic risk, the Indian government embarked upon a campaign of compulsory sterilization which was an egregious violation of human rights and Western governments supported population control throughout the developing world.

But it never happened. Ehrlich and others had not anticipated the Green Revolution and falling birth-rates.

And even at Oxford they make mistakes. Within days of issuing the Global Catastrophic Risk 2016 report, the experts were eating humble pie. A mathematician reviewed its calculations and concluded that "the Future of Humanity Institute seems very confused re: the future of humanity". The authors had to correct their most startling statistic. It doesn't inspire a lot of confidence in the ethics of existential risk.

Upsetting the balance of nature
MercatorNet, 22 January 2016

A British report on the irrelevance of "naturalness" could have far-reaching consequences.

It's not surprising that a report from the Nuffield Council on Bioethics, an influential independent British bioethics think tank, has received almost no publicity since its release last November. *"Ideas about naturalness in public and political debates about science, technology and medicine"* is not a title which sets the pulse racing.

Perhaps they should have christened it "Unnatural Acts". That would have guaranteed it blanket coverage in the London tabloids.

But this study of why people call some things "natural" or "unnatural" could be one of the most important position papers of the decade. It is fundamentally an attempt to deconstruct and then to outlaw what US bioethicist Leon Kass called "the wisdom of repugnance".

A new medical technology encounters the most resistance when voters describe it as "unnatural". If you nailed a placard to a door with the words "plague within", politicians could not run away fast enough. So one strategy to secure government approval for controversial new technologies is to reframe the debate -- either to make the technologies look natural or to send the word "naturalness" to Coventry. The latter is the approach favoured by the Nuffield Council.

As the report points out: "People's ideas about naturalness

may influence the degree to which advances in science, technology and medicine are embraced or opposed by the UK public." So it sets out to deconstruct the word, to make it meaningless, and so to bury it as a term of intellectual discourse. If people can be taught to distrust their own moral intuitions, securing regulatory approval for the most far-fetched projects will be a snap.

The British scientific establishment, which is fond of white papers, has a lot of experience in massaging public opinion. In recent years, it has shepherded through Parliament laws permitting "unnatural" technologies like IVF, mitochondrial donation, hybrid embryos, GM foods, animal experimentation, cloning, surrogacy, and gamete donation.

The most famous of all British white papers, the 1957 *Wolfenden Report on Homosexuality*, covered much the same ground when it concluded that homosexuality was neither a disease nor a crime. (A decade later the UK repealed its ban on homosexual offences.) Nor was homosexuality "unnatural", the committee argued, for the same reasons that the Nuffield Council was to employ 60 years later:

> Similarly, we have avoided the use of the terms "natural" and "unnatural" in relation to sexual behaviour, for they depend for their force upon certain explicit theological or philosophical interpretations, and without these interpretations their use imports an approving or a condemnatory note into a discussion where dispassionate thought and statement should not be hindered by adherence to particular preconceptions. (paragraph 36)

There in a nutshell is the Superior Man's case against the Common Man's wisdom of repugnance: only a philosopher can muddle this out and we are not the philosophical kind; the only good reason is: *does it do harm?*

Since philosophers have been debating naturalness for at least

2,400 years old, yet another committee of British panjandrums was unlikely light up the sky with intellectual fireworks. But their report has a more limited purpose: to give the government an arsenal of arguments to justify potentially controversial policies.

There is no better strategy for dismissing a moral argument than to say that it is meaningless, ambiguous and confusing. The words "human dignity" have already been expelled from the vocabulary of most bioethicists after being subjected to this sort of analysis. It also works for "naturalness".

The report sets out five understandings of *naturalness* that show the different ways in which the terms "natural" and "unnatural" are used:

> *Neutral*: a neutral/sceptical view that does not equate naturalness with goodness.
>
> *Wisdom of nature*: the idea that nature has found the correct or best ways of doing things and should not be "tampered" with.
>
> *God and religion*: the idea that certain technologies distort God's creation or go against the will of God.
>
> *Natural purpose*: the idea that living things have natural purpose, essence or functions which is linked to what is good for them and which science shouldn't seek to change.
>
> *Disgust and monstrosity*: a response of disgust, revulsion or fear prompted by novel technologies.

"It is too simplistic to suggest that natural things are good and unnatural things are bad, yet we see many examples of this being implied through the media, in advertising and on the packaging of many products we buy. Our findings show that people use the terms nature, natural and unnatural to express a range of values, beliefs, hopes and fears," said Roland Jackson, the chair of the naturalness project.

Amongst the recommendations made by the committee is some Orwellian finger-wagging at journalists, politicians, policy-makers, manufacturers and advertisers to mind their language. Tom Shakespeare, member of the Council's Steering Group, said: "The use of these words by journalists, politicians and others to convey a good or bad view of science is lazy and clichéd. People often have genuine concerns, beliefs and values which should be answered, not just dismissed. Everyone involved in key debates about science should avoid using these terms, unless they are willing to explore and engage with the hopes and fears that lie behind them".

From now on, in other words, the term "natural" is to be regarded as "doubleplusungood", as they used to say in 1984.

Although the report concludes that more precision in the use of the word "natural" will help people communicate more effectively, it's hard to escape the feeling that the British government has something up its sleeve. After all, it is not in the business of lexicography.

And it does. While the report is cautiously phrased, it prepares the ground for an official government stand that the word "natural" is so ambiguous and confusing that arguments based on "naturalness" carry no weight whatsoever. It's hard to imagine what cannot be approved in the new bio-technologies if this happens.

The same argument can be deployed in public policy arguments about sexual morality, just as the authors of the Wolfenden Report did 60 years ago. If "naturalness" is banned from public discourse, how can homosexuality, gay marriage or transgenderism be called wrong? Or, for that matter, incest or bestiality? Or human enhancement or genetic engineering? Or genetically modified animals or geo-engineering the climate?

The goal of Newspeak, the official language in George Orwell's *1984*, was to make negative thoughts literally unthinkable: "This was done partly by the invention of new words," he wrote, "but chiefly by eliminating undesirable words and by stripping such words as remained of unorthodox meanings, and so far as possible of all secondary meanings whatever."

Is this what the Nuffield Council has in mind?

Do zombies have human rights?

MercatorNet, 30 October 2012

How prepared are you for the moral dilemmas of a zombie apocalypse?

The approach of Halloween seems an appropriate time to raise the sensitive topic of zombie euthanasia. Of course, Halloween festivities may be muted on America's eastern seaboard. A once-in-a-generation storm, Hurricane Sandy, is lashing New York at the moment. Lights are off, streets are flooded, traffic has stopped. There may not be much trick-or-treating.

People who have been preparing for the zombie apocalypse are ready for scenarios like this. Last year the Centers for Disease Control and Prevention published a book "Preparedness 101: Zombie Pandemic" which tells you everything you need to know about coping with epidemics of infectious diseases -- hordes of flesh-eating zombies, for example. Hurricanes are a piece of cake compared to a zombie apocalypse.

Officials at Federal Emergency Management Agency (FEMA) believe that a zombie apocalypse is only a remote possibility on current trends, but it is not impossible. In fact, according to a survey carried out by the Committee to Re-elect President Obama, about 48% of Americans are already zombies. A poll commissioned by the Committee to elect Mitt Romney found that the figure is about 47%. Clearly, if either of these is correct, the price for unpreparedness could be high. The CDC's handbook should be in every home.

But one important issue which is not addressed in the CDC's

manual is whether or not it is ethical to euthanize zombies. George Romero's classic zombie documentaries, *Night of the Living Dead, Dawn of the Dead, Day of the Dead, Diary of the Dead, Survival of the Dead,* and so on, make some very big and very questionable ethical assumptions.

Much of the action is taken up with ingenious methods of dispatching zombies. But is it really morally permissible to kill them?

There are bioethicists who contend that it is. Kyle Munkittrick, of Pop Bioethics, has outlined three principles involved in deciding whether zombies may be ethically shot, pitchforked, beheaded, incinerated, etc: the dignity of the body, the state of the infection, and the zombie's potential for recovering consciousness.

Dignity of the body: a zombie has none. De-animating a zombie restores its dignity. "Therefore, it is acceptable to lobotomize, ignite, and/or puree the zombie without violating your Kantian commitment to the dignity of the body."

The state of the infection. The situations of people who have been recently infected, who are in transition to zombiehood, or who are fully-committed zombies are different. But the safest course of action is immediate euthanasia.

Consciousness. Even if zombichood is reversible, the person would survive with significant neurological deficits which would compromise its dignity. The safest course of action is immediate euthanasia.

However, this is a shabby utilitarian approach to decision-making which assumes (a) that the zombies are really dead and (b) that they are no longer humans. If either of these are false, the case for a utilitarian solution to the zombie apocalypse collapses.

Let's examine whether they are really dead.

A professor at Harvard Medical School, Steven Schlozman, has just published a book on the neuroanatomy of the zombie brain, *The Zombie Autopsies*, to help prepare for the possibility of a zombie apocalypse. In a very informative video, "Zombie Autopies 101", he dissects a brain to show the parts which are malfunctioning.

A zombie's shambling gait is due to problems with its cerebellum. A zombie craves human flesh because its ventromedial hypothalamus is "messed up". It is stupid because its frontal lobe has been damaged, perhaps irretrievably. its rage is due to a malfunctioning amygdala. The only way to kill zombies is to crush the brain stem, destroying their autonomic nervous system and making it impossible for their hearts to beat or for them to breathe. A meat cleaver in the frontal lobe or parietal lobe may not be sufficient disrupt their functioning.

The conclusion to be drawn from this data is that the zombies are not dead. They are not even brain-dead. Neuroscientists at the University of California San Francisco have identified the particular disease: Consciousness Deficit Hypoactivity Disorder. Victims suffer from "the loss of rational, voluntary and conscious behaviour replaced by delusional/impulsive aggression, stimulus-driven attention, and the inability to coordinate motor or linguistic behaviours".

So, while they may be different from the rest of us, there is no reason why these differences should not be respected and why their constitutional rights should be ignored. They are still human, albeit severely impaired and very hungry.

One of the main insights of another documentary investigation of the zombie condition, *Shaun of the Dead*, is that a very thin line separates the day-to-day life of zombies and aimless inner city dwellers who spend their lives watching television and tossing back beers.

In fact, the documentary shows that it may be possible for zombies to regain some cognitive capacity and to live normal lives (as long as they are chained up). The final scene depicts life after the apocalypse. One of the zombies, Ed, has been domesticated and plays video games in a shed in his friend's backyard – which is not much different from his pre-zombified occupations.

It could even be argued that zombification is an enhanced form of humanity. Although a significant amount of cognitive capacity is sacrificed, zombies gain in strength and endurance. Life is also less complicated by existential anxieties when the daily grind is focused solely upon the next meal. Some people might actually prefer to live as zombies.

Self-preservation is deemed ethical by most reputable bioethicists. Consequently, in the midst of the mayhem of a zombie apocalypse, there can be no objection to killing zombies, provided that it is done humanely.

The question of euthanasia arises after the zombies have been beaten back and the infection placed under control. What should be done with the surviving zombies? Given the successful outcome for Ed in *Shaun of the Dead*, perhaps we could think of innovative ways to house zombies and integrate them back into society. As long as there is no danger of infecting less impaired humans, they could play with X-Boxes or watch reruns of "Seinfeld".

Mars Mission Bioethics 101

Australasian Science, December 2014

> *A one-way trip to Mars, funded from the rights to a reality TV show, raises many bioethical issues.*

All Trekkies are familiar with unavoidable ethical dilemmas in deep space. A Dutch group called Mars One is seeking to create them by sending four volunteers to establish a settlement on Mars in April 2023. It will be a one-way trip.

A number of big technology companies are interested in contributing to Mars One and some big names are publicising it. Gerard 't Hooft, a Dutch Nobel laureate in physics, says: "This project seems to me to be the only way to fulfil dreams of mankind's expansion into space."

The latest plan is for a crew of four to leave in 2024 and to land in 2025. Thereafter crews will leave every two years to build up the colony. The first mission will cost an estimated US$6 billion; later missions only $4 billion.

How will such an expensive and risky project be financed? With revenues from reality TV. Paul Römer, the Dutch inventor of *Big Brother*, is a big fan: "This mission to Mars can be the biggest media event in the world. Reality meets talent show with no ending and the whole world watching."

The TV series will begin with the selection of the astronauts. "Because this mission is humankind's mission, Mars One has the intention to make this a democratic decision," says the company. "The whole world will have a vote which group of four will be the first humans on Mars."

The list of bioethical issues with this project is very long. The first is whether it is ethical to send people on a one-way trip. Is it exploration or suicide? The Mars One website invokes Australian history to defend the idea: "thousands of Europeans agreed to do just that – they took all they owned and moved to Australia, for example. That agreement did not come with a return ticket."

But there are many other issues as well.

Lifeboat dilemmas. What happens if an accident reduces the amount of air or other resources for a four-man flight to two or three? Should the astronauts draw straws to decide which one should die? Should they kill the astronaut who adds the least value to the mission?

Pregnancies in space. Sexual tension makes for good TV, so the "whole world" might vote to send two men and two women into space. The company advises its astronauts not to have children for the time being until some of the technical issues are solved, but it says nothing about sex. A space child could be seriously handicapped because of space radiation and micro-gravity during the flight and on Mars. Will abortions be performed in space? Will astronauts be sterilized before leaving?

Privacy. The astronauts' every action will be monitored for their whole lives. It's impossible to test the psychological pressure on the astronauts here on Earth.

Bad technical planning. Researchers at MIT released a scathing feasibility study of Mars One in September. They claimed that if all food is grown inside the settlement, the vegetation would produce so much oxygen that the colonists would suffocate. And with today's technology they could not produce enough water from the Martian soil.

Bad financial planning. What if the company backing

the trip runs out of money and cannot afford to resupply the station or bring the astronauts back home? As Karl D. Stephan, an engineering ethicist, commented: "Even the most debauched reality-TV shows up to now have not proposed to show us live scenes of slow starvation, but that's what we'd be dealing with. What would the dying colonists be thinking?"

Bad marketing planning. The day-to-day experience of trip to Mars and life on Mars will be about as exciting as watching paint dry. Will reality TV fans tune in? There was a great surge of interest after Apollo 11's crew, Neil Armstrong and Buzz Aldrin, walked on the Moon in 1969. But who remembers Apollo 12? Ominously, the other mission that kept people glued to their TV sets was Apollo 13, the near miss. Mars One's ratings will soar if the colonists are dying – but is it ethical to subject them to such risks?

A German astronaut who worked on the Space Shuttle, Ulrich Walter, believes that the project is too dangerous. "They make their money with that [TV] show," he told a newspaper. "They don't care what happens to those people in space."

Notwithstanding these problems – most of them quite obvious after a moment's reflection – 200,000 people applied for Mars One.

www.ingramcontent.com/pod-product-compliance
Lightning Source LLC
Chambersburg PA
CBHW021756230426
43669CB00006B/91